"A spectacular, state-of-the-art explanation of how magnetic therapy can relieve pain and promote healing."
—*Professor Alan Bennett, Kings College Medical School, London*

"Finally, a book about the future of drugless medicine— magnets and electromagnetic therapy. Thank you, Dr. Lawrence!"
—*James Coburn*

"Dr. Lawrence brought magnet therapy to my attention, for which I thank him."
—*Andy Griffith*

"Our research has confirmed that magnetic fields can have important effects on nerve growth and regeneration, and may provide other rewards, as clearly outlined in this useful book."
—*Betty Sisken, Ph.D., professor at the Center for Biomedical Engineering, University of Kentucky; president-elect, The Bioelectromagnetics Society*

"Dr. Rosch is probably the world's leading authority on stress."
—*Konstantin Sudakov, M.D., president, The Russian Academy of Sciences*

(more)

# Magnet Therapy

# Magnet Therapy

*The Pain Cure
Alternative*

RON LAWRENCE, M.D., PH.D.,
PAUL ROSCH, M.D., F.A.C.P.,
AND JUDITH PLOWDEN

**PRIMA HEALTH**
A Division of Prima Publishing

PRIMA HEALTH and colophon are trademarks of Prima Communications, Inc.

Prima Publishing has designed this book to provide information in regard to the subject matter covered. It is sold with the understanding that the publisher and the author are not liable for the misconception or misuse of information provided. Every effort has been made to make this book as complete and as accurate as possible. The purpose of this book is to educate. The author and Prima Publishing shall have neither liability nor responsibility to any person or entity with respect to any loss, damage, or injury caused or alleged to be caused directly or indirectly by the information contained in this book. The information presented herein is in no way intended as a substitute for medical counseling.

*Illustrations by Lisa Cooper*

**Library of Congress Cataloging-in-Publication Data**

Lawrence, Ron.
Magnet therapy : the pain cure alternative / by Ron Lawrence,
Paul Rosch, Judith Plowden.
p. cm.
Includes index.
ISBN 0-7615-1547-X
1. Magnetotherapy—Popular works.
I. Rosch, Paul. II. Plowden, Judith. III. Title.
RM893.L38 1998
615.8'45—dc21 98-12167
CIP
98 99 00 01 02 HH 10 9 8 7 6 5 4 3
Printed in the United States of America

**How to Order**
Single copies may be ordered from Prima Publishing, P.O. Box 1260BK, Rocklin, CA 95677; telephone (916) 632-4400. Quantity discounts are also available. On your letterhead, include information concerning the intended use of the books and the number of books you wish to purchase.

**Visit us online at www.primahealth.com**

*To our wives,*
*Eleanor Lawrence and Marguerite Rosch,*
*with thanks for their patience and support*
*during the writing of this book.*

# CONTENTS

# FOREWORD

Discovery: To increase our understanding of the world we live in and, thereby, to expand our individual reality is one of the greatest joys of being human. Another joy is sharing the fruits of discovery and knowledge with others. In all of human history there has never been a time of such exciting new discoveries as the one we live in. I have been privileged to participate in some of the great explorations of this century including a visit to our nearest planetary neighbor, the moon.

The ultimate goal of all explorers is to better understand oneself and one's relationship to the larger reality of the universe. This is no less true of the scientist in the laboratory than it is for the space explorer. From ancient to modern times, those who have explored the deeper mysteries of human processes share the same goal. And, often a new discovery appears quite unexpectedly.

During my journey aboard *Apollo 14,* I discovered that the universe is not composed of separate and discrete parts as described by our classical science, but is a universe of interconnected processes that can only be described as intelligent. This amazing and puzzling experience led me to found the Institute of Noetic Sciences in order to engage in full-time study of the "mind/body" problem. Eleven years would pass, however, before quantum science decisively demonstrated that all particles in the universe maintain a quantum interconnection that transcends classical notions of space and time. This interconnectedness is called non-locality. It would require twenty-five years before science demonstrated that this quantum correlation subtly operates through resonance to affect our everyday reality— even our perceptions—to produce effects previously considered mystical.

Knowledge of how our bodies operate has been teased slowly from nature—by tribal shamans and medicine men, and in modern times by physical, medical, and psychological scientists. The ancients knew more about the interconnectedness of things and methods of herbal and ritual healing that are only now being confirmed in principle by frontier physical and medical scientists. The problem has been that for over a century Western scientific thought has focused upon a chemical model of how the molecules, tissues, and organs of our bodies are organized and function. However, this biochemical model must be expanded to deeper levels in order to include the electromagnetic and quantum processes that play a major role in how nature (our bodies are an evolutionary product of nature) has organized itself.

Science makes progress by creating models (hypotheses) of nature, then testing our human experiences against these models. Only when an overwhelming preponderance of evidence suggests that certain experiences cannot be explained by the existing model do we reluctantly (often angrily and self righteously) abandon our cherished hypotheses. Most often it requires an overarching or meta-model that includes the previous model in some form. That is to say that nature consists of processes within processes within processes and our understanding of these processes must be consistent and complete at all levels and scales if our overall understanding is to be complete. And so it is with physical, chemical, biochemical, and electromagnetic and quantum theories. Each is more perplexing than the previous, but none by itself tells the whole story, as our bodies function on all these levels simultaneously.

Medical scientists have been investigating electrical, magnetic, and now electromagnetic and quantum influences on bodily functioning for several decades, but without widespread acceptance of their findings. The preponderance of evidence that magnetic fields can relieve pain in the body is sufficiently overwhelming that a major effort is now being mounted to discover how and why this is so. In order to understand all the subtle therapies that are now used in classical and contemporary medicine, we must first understand the electromagnetic properties, and then, the quantum properties of our bodies. This book tells us about some of that effort.

I have been privileged to know and work with the authors of this book and other researchers cited herein. I have followed the pioneering work of Dr. Robert Becker for over twenty-five years. Dr. Paul Rosch and I have been not only professional colleagues but occasional golfing partners as well. Dr. Rosch introduced me to Dr. Ron Lawrence at a medical conference. The progress of these dedicated pioneers to discover new modalities of health and healing is impressive and will require much effort and a number of years before the complete picture emerges of how nature has used basic physical, chemical, electromagnetic, and quantum energies in

building our bodies and minds. Only then will humankind
have all the tools to relieve suffering and to create more positive lives.

—Edgar Mitchell, Sc.D.
astronaut, *Apollo 14*

# ACKNOWLEDGMENTS

We are especially grateful to Julian Plowden for his editorial eye, and for the technical assistance of Dr. Marko Markov.

We thank our invaluable assistants: Cindy Kornspan, Cheryl Brown, Jennifer Gassett, and James Reagan.

Special thanks to Brenda Nichols and Jamie Miller of Prima for their tireless work in making this book a reality.

# INTRODUCTION

Imagine how it was, living thousands of years ago when science and technology were still far in the future. We observed the forces of the universe at work. We saw that all objects, light or heavy, eventually fell to earth; that everything, if one could cut it apart, seemed to be made of ever-smaller other things; that when the gods were angry, lightning came from the sky, and that strange stones could attract or repel each other or cause metal objects to move. We observed all these forces of the universe with wonder and awe, but the last one was on a scale we could handle—a magic our children could play with.

Our early ancestors didn't have the devices we now use to peer into the intimate life of the atom. They could only observe phenomena, not measure them; and they observed another force. They called it by various names, and imagined it was the invisible force of life itself. It keeps our hearts beating, our lungs drawing in air, our brains sparking with ideas. Without this fundamental energy, there is no life. So, they speculated, could it be related to the other invisible force of the magic stones?

Since the breakthrough theories of Einstein and other physicists, we now have terms for the four forces in the universe:

the weak nuclear force, the strong nuclear force, gravity, and the electromagnetic.

All our body cells have some energy or force flowing through them. To wax poetic for a moment, we are not only "such stuff that dreams are made of," but we are also the dust of ancient stars, and in that dust there are tiny magnetic particles.

Atoms, cells, human beings, the earth—all are charged with magnetic energy. So are the push and pull of weather patterns in the hemispheres, the movement of sun and stars. If you think about it, the whole universe is magnetic. Including perhaps the attraction between two lovers, which once was credited solely to "chemistry." The old cliché "opposites attract" governs the fact that all opposites are dynamic, creating change, powering life forward. Yin and yang, hot and cold, dark and light. By day, the positive field from the sun; by night, the negative field of the earth.

Although magnetic therapy believers and skeptics may be poles apart (sorry!) they are alive to argue the matter solely because all humans function by the same invisible life force the ancients instinctively knew. The Chinese call it *Qi,* to the Japanese it is *chi,* in Sanskrit it is *prana.* This flow of invisible life force energy, circulating through the body in an orderly prescribed fashion through pathways called meridians, guides the science of acupuncture, a therapy from China now officially accepted in the West. The ancient practice of yoga is based on energy centers called *chakras* at sites up the spinal column to the top of the head. Similar channels were called *nadis* in Sanskrit and *Tsas* in Tibetan. It was believed that illness occurred when the flow, or communication, through these pathways was blocked and/or the supply of energy became deficient.

Did the ancients know more than we ever suspected? Why is it that the magnetic force seems to influence the channels of the life energy, or *Qi,* as in acupuncture, and relieves pain? There is a strong element of magic in this interaction. And what is the force at work when a natural healer lays on hands or directs thoughts at a sick patient? *Kirlian* photography has captured a blazing aura that cannot be explained by scientists. And sometimes, to everyone's amazement, this type of healing succeeds.

The fascination of magic lies in the apparent suspension of the laws of Nature. We humans observe a natural phenomenon, marvel at it, learn to make use of it, and then attempt to explain how and why. Over the centuries, explanations fall by the way as theories are disproved and discarded, or simply get shot down. Sometimes science, each specialty with its own focus and agenda, finds itself playing catch-up with the phenomenon.

## Twin Aspects of the Same Force

As to the electromagnetic force, humans by now have acquired a great deal of knowledge about the electro aspect. Electricity has given us many of the technological marvels and benefits of the modern era. The magnetic component has produced devices that power motors, radio, television, and computers, to name just a few, but even as our scientific knowledge of electricity grew, it didn't penetrate as far into the magnetic aspect. Because everyone knew that it existed but couldn't be truly explained, in the past it was sometimes exploited by charlatans, and this has tended to overshadow its healing potential.

Critics need to be convinced by solid data on why and how magnetic therapy works. Modern medicine already uses some forms of this energy for diagnosis (MRI: magnetic resonance imaging) and healing (mending bone fractures more quickly with electromagnetic fields).

The two medical applications are closely related because of the almost-twin aspects of the same force. All magnets can produce an electric current. A magnet placed in a coil when moving induces a current of electricity in the coil and vice versa. Take a coil carrying electricity, put iron inside it, and you make it magnetic. You are probably familiar with the electrocardiogram (ECG) and electroencephalogram (EEG) as used in modern medicine. These same measurements can be taken in magnetic values, in the magnetocardiogram and magneto-encephalography. Awfully big words, but you'll see how these forces constantly overlap. In this book, we will try to simplify by focusing on permanent magnets, but will sometimes refer to electromagnetic therapy as well. What is important is that the preservation and balance of magnetic fields in the human body can be facilitated with permanent magnets.

## Magnetic Therapy Already Popular

Today, magnets are expanding their role into the world of health and healing, offering dramatic pain relief. As a healing therapy, magnetism has taken off like a rocket, especially in the popular arena. The sales of magnets are growing exponentially. It is claimed that permanent magnets have sold over $2 billion last year worldwide, mostly for use against pain. Famous sports figures and senior golfers are among those who praise magnets for stopping aches and soreness, plus giving a vital energy lift. As people everywhere begin to seek the power of natural forms of healing, they find magnets are versatile and safe tools to help the body's healing process. People are inevitably drawn to a natural therapy that is safe, noninvasive, inexpensive, non-addictive, and produces no side effects which are often seen with drugs.

Magnetic therapy is well advanced in Japan, China, India, Australia, and Germany. Here in the United States, however, the majority of physicians have been slow to recognize and embrace it.

What science and medicine are trying to do at this time is pin down the "how" and the "why." Exactly how do magnetic fields act within the body? Why do they relieve pain? Many researchers believe that permanent magnets increase circulation, energizing and oxygenating the blood, and that this increased blood flow stimulates the body's own natural healing process. Still, with so many different applications and mechanisms, magnetic therapy seems to resist precise explanation of the sort that satisfies the stringent requirements of scientific research—funding from major medical centers and double-blind studies published in peer-reviewed journals. But as you will see in this book, slowly but surely the mysterious force is beginning to yield its secrets.

Public demand forces change. You can be sure that in the days ahead magnetic therapy will be the subject of much heated discussion and controversy.

The applications for magnetic therapy make an impressive list, ranging from arthritis to wound healing, nerve injury, carpal tunnel syndrome, and headaches. New applications have been announced at recent conferences, such as for the painful disease known as fibromyalgia, and Attention Deficit Disorder, so widespread in American school-age children. Some of the symptoms of stress, the unwanted side effect of our fast-lane lifestyles, can be stopped by magnetic therapy. Above all, pain *can be* alleviated.

Magnets are a godsend for chronic pain, and we will explore this fully. Indeed, you may have been irresistibly attracted to this book because you are one of the millions who suffer some form of chronic pain. Magnetic fields in their many forms can help promote both pain relief and healing. We will try to explain how magnets work as clearly and simply as possible. Because we hope many health professionals will be encouraged to look further into this remarkable method of therapy, we urge you to share this book with your doctor. That is why you may find some sections a little too technical, or filled with medical terms. Feel free to skip them, but they will help to convince your doctor that this is a valid therapy.

Most physicians are understandably skeptical about recent claims that magnetic therapies can be so successful. Doctors also have very justifiable concerns that seriously ill patients, caught up in the current enthusiasm for alternative medicine, might bypass a treatment that could be life-saving in certain situations. On the other hand, there are very well-documented case histories that are hard to dispute. This is particularly true for some now being related, in growing numbers, by physicians who started out as skeptics. To the remaining skeptics, even careful evaluation of improved patients meets with the dismissal that it must be due to the power of suggestion, or some sort of placebo effect. But how can the effect in animals and babies be explained as placebo? And, ultimately, who cares, if magnets can relieve pain and other problems?

Therapy with permanent magnets is where acupuncture was thirty years ago. What was considered frivolous then is even being paid for today by the seriously profit-oriented health insurance companies. Some preposterous claims have been made for magnetic therapy, giving rise to confusion. But while scientists seek (and regulators demand) precise and clear demonstrations of truth, complete with statistics, pain sufferers are seeking relief, and are using magnets by the millions. The greater millions who don't yet know about magnets should have the information for the sake of their health, for pain relief and all the other uses of magnetic therapy. Everyone deserves clear explanations and scientific backup, not the often-confusing exaggerations found on the Internet and from other sources. In this book you will find the experience of two medical doctors who, almost despite themselves, became interested in magnets for healing, and have used them on family, friends, and numerous patients.

Both doctors believe in the need for proper studies to prove a procedure or a substance is both effective and safe. It's important to remember that such studies can cost a great deal of money, which is one reason why new therapies and natural nutrients that can't be patented take so long to become approved and accepted. Everything gets started somewhere, and the value of patient anecdotes and small case studies from individual doctors should not be thrown out by mainstream medicine. It is this route that a new therapy must take as it begins to be noticed, tested, and finally accepted.

The extraordinary thing about this book is that the authors are two mainstream medical doctors with solid academic credentials and decades of clinical experience, who are deeply involved in a therapy still on the fringes.

Dr. Lawrence says:

> When it comes to new health trends, I consider myself pretty
> old-fashioned, a practitioner of orthodox Western medicine
> who happens to be open-minded, who has tried many

modalities. Surgery saves lives, and I wouldn't be without medications for certain emergencies. But I would find it beneficial to be able to give lower dosages of most drugs to my patients, and magnets can help me do this. If I had to go and stay on a desert island, the only health items I would take would be morphine, digitalis, aspirin, and epinephrine. *Plus magnets.*

Dr. Rosch is equally conservative, and cites Santayana's credo:

Skepticism is the chastity of the mind. Do not surrender it to the first comer.

On the other hand, he feels that you need to keep an open mind. He is equally convinced that magnets can relieve pain and provide other benefits, and feels that most doctors don't share this opinion because of arrogance or ignorance. Hopefully, this book will help to open minds that have been shut tight.

Both doctors believe that a greater understanding of how magnets work may provide important insights into communication pathways in the body. Such information could explain widely accepted but poorly understood matters such as the placebo effect, and the ability of a firm faith and strong social support to improve health by reducing stress.

We hope you will find great rewards in learning more about magnetic fields and their role in optimal health. Magnets have *no* side effects as many drugs do. Magnets *can* relieve pain. Magnets speed up the body's natural healing processes. No matter what side of the fence you're on, no matter whether the finer points of the how and the why are still being debated, magnets work. They represent a modern use of ancient wisdom.

If you have come this far, then take the next step, into a world of magic and healing—the world of magnets, powered by man's undying curiosity, from the simple wonder of the ancients to the leading edge of today's technology.

# CHAPTER 1

# Following the Magnetic Trail

- Paracelsus
- The Doctor of Animal Magnetism
- Explorations into Electromagnetism
- Magnets Come to America
- A Short History of Medicine

Exploration of magnetism in the past few centuries is a colorful story, complete with eccentric characters. But only a few legends and writings have come down to us from our early ancestors who found and used the magnetic force—mainly from China, India, Egypt, and Greece.

Long before the existence of any known writings, a well-developed system of medicine existed in China based on the premise that health depended on the circulation of vital energies in the body through prescribed pathways (see figure 1.1). In Chinese medicine, this internal strength was called *Qi (chi),* and was derived from two opposing influences: yin and yang. Illness resulted when these were not balanced, the natural flow of *Qi* was blocked, or there was some disturbance in the normal equilibrium between this energy and forces found in Nature.

Then came the written word. *The Yellow Emperor's Book of Internal Medicine,* the earliest written record of medicine, dating all the way back to 2000 B.C., describes how such imbalances could be corrected by means of acupuncture, moxibustion (heat), and application of magnetic stones at specific sites. We can assume that these recommendations were based on supportive evidence that had accumulated over previous centuries. Inserting needles and applying heat are understandable, since these can be felt. But why would anyone be prompted to try stones with magnetic properties that could not be sensed? The most likely explanation is that the ancient Chinese were impressed by the magnet's apparent ability to cause objects to move, possibly signifying that they also possessed some potent life force that could be utilized to fortify human *Qi* (see figures 1.2 and 1.3).

The ancient religious scriptures of the Hindus, known as the Vedas, also believed to be 4,000 years old, mention the treatment of disease with *ashmana* and *siktavati,* "instruments of stone," which were almost certainly lodestones. In India there was a belief that a dying person should be positioned in the bed with the head toward the north and feet pointing south, to induce magnetic harmony between earth and body. This was meant to ease pain and soothe the departing spirit. To this day, many people in India believe the north–south position is best for sleeping at night.

The most popular magnet legend is that a young Greek shepherd named Magnes, in a region called Magnesia, first

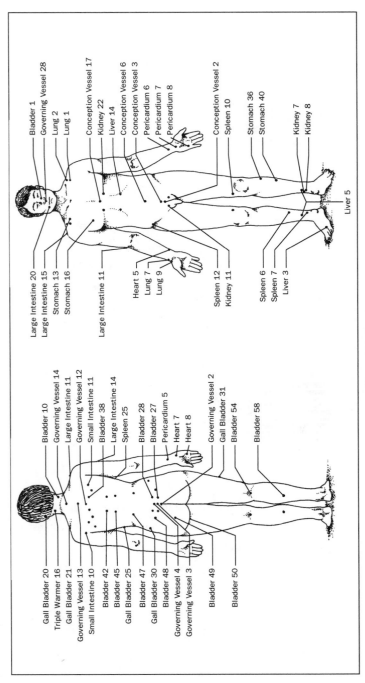

**Figure 1.1**

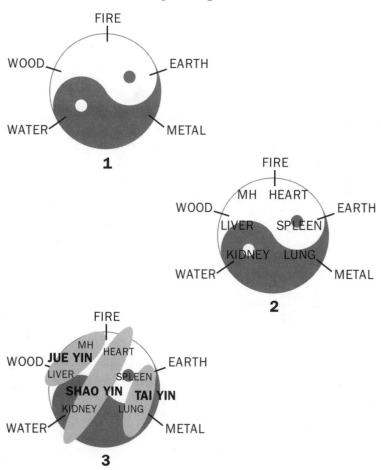

**Figure 1.2**

*Qi* contains both *yin* and *yang* (1). Each of these are linked to different elements and organs (2). These, in turn, are associated with other characteristics.

There are also energy axes consisting of two organs and their sphere of influence with two poles that represent the element qualities, as well as the *yin* and *yang* characteristics of their organs (3).

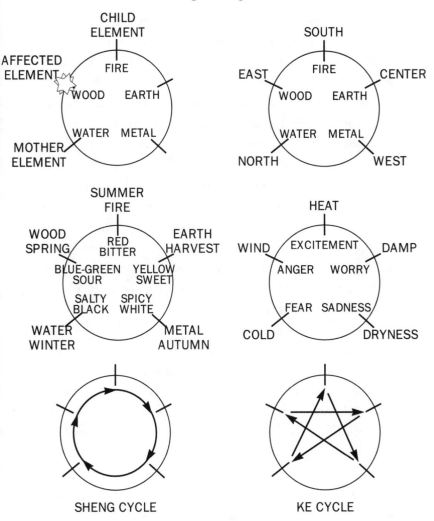

**Figure 1.3**

*Yin* and *yang* are represented in varying degrees in everything including people, organs, elements, direction, season, color, taste, climate, and emotions. Each of these attributes is also interrelated to each other. During health, all of these are kept in balance by an orderly flow of *Qi*. This is regulated by the *Sheng Cycle* of evolution and the energy dynamics of the *Ke Cycle* of control or transformation.

discovered the powerful pull between his iron staff, the nails of his shoes, and a nearby magnetic lodestone. This tale shows you how legends can become embellished in the telling. If indeed there was a young shepherd, his staff was almost certainly made of wood. Perhaps all that happened was that he was surprised to find small stones clinging to the iron nails in his shoes. However, Pliny the Elder is said to have firmly believed in the legend.

Large accumulations of magnetite or magnetic oxide were referred to by the ancient Greeks as live-stones *(lapis vivus)*, since they moved for no visible reason when placed close together, and would also attract anything containing iron. Magnet is said to be derived from *Magnes lithos,* "stone from Magnesia," a region rich in magnetic stones, which later became *magneta* in Latin.

Then in the seventh century B.C., the Greek philosopher and mathematician Thales noted that amber, which was fossilized tree resin used to make beads, also had the power of attraction. If amber was rubbed with a piece of wool, it would pick up light objects such as feathers, straw, or dried grass, but not iron or other metals. We know now that he was describing static electricity. Thales concluded that rubbing the amber imparted some human energy that had now made it magnetic. He said the magnet (lodestone) "has soul because it attracts iron." And he also said, "All things are full of gods."

Egyptian physicians ascribed a variety of therapeutic effects to lodestones. Another legend claims that Queen Cleopatra of Egypt wore a small magnet as an amulet on her forehead to preserve her youth. How did Cleopatra know this was a shrewd move? The pineal gland, a tiny gland in the shape of a pine nut (hence the name), is located behind the forehead in the center of the brain. We still have much to learn about melatonin and the pineal, but we do know that electromagnetic fields can affect pineal function. Melatonin, which is secreted at night by the pineal gland, is a powerful antioxidant with potential anti-aging properties.

There is good evidence from human, animal, and bacterial studies that the body's orientation to the earth's magnetic poles can influence behavior and physiology. And melatonin has become an extremely popular sleep aid, effective in jetlag, and as an anti-aging supplement.

The power of lodestones also may have been known in ancient Tibet. Still today, Tibetan monks use bar magnets placed on the skull in accordance with a particular protocol for improving the concentration and learning capabilities of beginning monks.

In the early days of Rome, electromagnetism was used in a rather odd way. Some Roman physicians used the charge from electric eels to treat arthritis and gout.

In medieval times in Europe, we find doctors reporting that magnets could cure not only arthritis and gout, but also conditions such as melancholy, baldness, and some poisonings. And during all these centuries, on the other side of the planet, the Chinese were using magnets to assist in navigation.

# Paracelsus

Let us fast forward through the long Dark Ages, complete with horrible plagues, when life was "nasty, brutish, and short" to a physician born in Switzerland the year after Columbus discovered America. Paracelsus was his name. He brought medicine forward by advancing the concept of disease, rather than the reigning theory of illness being due to disturbances in the body's "humors." The concept of the four "humors" had previously been promoted by Greek physician Galen (A.D. 130–200) and accepted as dogma.

Paracelsus gained fame as a remarkable physician, but was also skilled in chemistry and metallurgy. During his stormy career, he discovered and used the healing powers of the magnet. He was an eccentric fellow with a huge ego matched by a brilliant, creative mind. Some say he was the inspiration for the story of Dr. Faust, who sold his soul to the devil.

He was christened Philippus Aureolus Theophrastus Bombastus von Hohenheim. (It's understandable that he later changed a name like that!) He chose Paracelsus to acknowledge his debt to Celsus, the Roman physician and author of *De Re Medecina,* one of the first books published after the invention of the printing press, and our major source of information on early Greek and Roman medicine.

He detested Galen as a fraud, and believed that illness resulted from external agents that attacked the body. For example, he pronounced that lung problems of miners resulted from tiny particles of minerals in the mine itself rather than the evil intent of mountain spirits.

Paracelsus was the first to recognize a hereditary pattern in syphilis, the association of cretinism with endemic goiter, and the paralysis that sometimes followed head injuries. He advocated the use of mercury, sulfur, iron, arsenic, and other chemicals to fight different disease-causing agents. He also provided the basis for modern homeopathy, by proposing that some diseases could be cured by minuscule doses of "similars," or substances that could produce similar symptoms.

While Paracelsus knew nothing about the Chinese concept of *Qi,* he too believed that some ethereal, esoteric force in nature could energize people. He wrote that this internal energy was pervasive, unifying body and mind, and that although the body consisted of many separate parts, all parts influenced one another.

He wrote:

"The power to see does not come from the eye, the power to hear does not come from the ear, nor the power to feel from the nerves; but it is the spirit of man that sees through the eyes, hears through the ears, and feels by means of the nerves. Wisdom and reason and thought are not contained in the brain, but belong to the invisible and universal spirit which feels through the heart and thinks through the brain."

He also stated:

"Even the ignorant know that man has a heart and lungs, brain and stomach; but he thinks that each of these organs are separate and independent things that have nothing to do with each other."

In the healthy person, he believed, these structures acted in synergy, so that the total effect was greater than the sum of their individual contributions. Not only was there no separation of mind and body but, Paracelsus believed, thoughts or feelings could produce physical effects. Thus he anticipated, by four hundred years, the concepts of holistic and psychosomatic medicine, psychoneuroimmunology, and the placebo effect.

According to Paracelsus,

"The spirit is the master, the imagination is the instrument, the body is the plastic material. The moral atmosphere surrounding the patient can have a strong influence on the course of his disease. It is not the curse or blessing that

works, but the idea. The imagination produces the effect . . .
To think is to act on the plane of thought, and if the
thought is intense enough, it may produce an effect on the
physical plane."

The glue that binds all the different parts of the body
together, and the medium through which their effects were
made manifest, was this mysterious life force. Paracelsus called
it *archaeus,* from the Greek word for ancient, or first. Much like
*Qi,* it might be replenished by natural energies found in certain
herbs and foods. However, Paracelsus believed that *archaeus* was
most influenced by the mysterious force found in magnets,
which could energize the body and promote self-healing. He
proclaimed that all inflammations and many diseases could be
cured by magnetism, better than by means of any medicine. As
the psychiatrist Carl Jung wrote, "We see in Paracelsus not only
a pioneer in the domains of chemical medicine, but also in
those of an empirical psychological healing science."

Where did this *archaeus* energy so essential for life originate? Paracelsus explained that "the human body is a vapour,
materialized by sunshine mixed with the stars." This melds
rather nicely with the most popular theory of the origin of the
universe—that all matter and energy came from the "big
bang." We know now that all life on earth evolved under the
influence of persistent and powerful environmental magnetic
forces, and the earth itself is a giant magnet. Scientists have
just discovered that its inner core, which is a molten iron mass
1,500 miles wide and heavier than the moon, is spinning independently and slightly faster than the revolution of the planet
itself. This helps to explain the changes in the earth's magnetic field that have taken place over long periods of time,
including a periodic reversal of its magnetic poles.

Strictly speaking, all matter seems to be magnetic. Physicists can measure the magnetic properties of salt, glass, plastic, copper, and living tissue with sufficiently sensitive devices. Each of us has magnetic energy characteristics that not only differ between individuals, but may vary in different parts of the body, as well as with changing states of health. Although Paracelsus didn't know any of this, he was firmly convinced of the power of magnets, and the ability of magnetism to replenish *archaeus* energy and to correct disorders due to *archaeus* energy deficiency.

Magnets had traditionally been employed by physicians to retrieve shattered arrowheads, parts of knives, and other iron foreign bodies embedded in tissues. Paracelsus also used magnets to treat everything from diarrhea and epilepsy to various types of hemorrhage. Lodestones were ground up to make powders that could be applied as a magnetic salve, or ingested, and quack medicinal applications of magnets quickly became popular.

But Paracelsus was not popular with everyone. His brilliance, ego, violent temper, and contempt for other scientists meant that he walked alone. He died mysteriously in Salzburg, Austria, at the age of 48, possibly at the hands of his enemies.

Magnets also generated great interest because the compass had now made it possible to more accurately establish trade routes and explore the world than was possible by steering ships based on the position of certain stars. As we noted, the Chinese were the first to discover this; but centuries later, Christopher Columbus and others observed that the magnetic north of the compass was not the true north according to the stars, and that this magnetic deviation also varied in different parts of the world. Equally curious was the fact that all magnets had two opposite poles at their ends. The ends of magnets that faced the same way would repel each other if you tried to push them together, but opposite poles strongly attracted one another. In addition, if you kept cutting a magnet in two, these two opposite poles persisted, no matter how small the resultant segment. It was also difficult to explain how magnets could cause iron filings to move, even though they were separated by pieces of paper, or how ordinary iron could be temporarily magnetized to behave like a permanent magnet.

All of these magnetic phenomena were intensively investigated and clarified at the turn of the sixteenth century by William Gilbert, a mathematician who became a prosperous London physician, even attending Queen Elizabeth I and James I. He debunked lodestone salves and powders, pointing out that only the stone, which he found to be "beneficial in many diseases of the human system," could attract iron. (He did not know that most of the iron in the body is found in hemoglobin, which is essential for carrying oxygen to all cells.) He also demonstrated that steel retains its magnetism better than iron, and that there was a difference between magnetism and the static electricity that developed when amber was rubbed. He called this "electrica," from *èlektron,* the Greek word for amber, and showed that other substances could also produce this effect. He is credited as the first to see electricity and magnetism as separate forces.

In his major writing, *De Magnete,* he explained the variable magnetic deviation of compasses in different parts of the world, the inclination to a vertical position when a magnet was not in a horizontal plane, and the revolution of the earth in relation to the stars. This work was published in 1600, shortly after England had defeated the invincible Spanish Armada. It was Gilbert who proposed for the first time that the earth was actually a large lodestone. We could update that to: The earth is a huge magnet. In his Latin it goes: "Magnus magnes ipse est globus terrestris."

Queen Elizabeth I, who had a strong interest in science, supported Gilbert. With her keen mind she recognized that navigation would play an important role in commerce, establishing new colonies, and maintaining the supremacy of her fleet.

Gilbert's explorations into the medical and scientific uses of magnetic energy had a powerful influence. A magnetic cure for strangulated hernia was developed, in which patients were fed iron filings, and the trapped intestine was freed from the surrounding sheath of tissues by the external application of a strong magnet.

By the middle 1700s, more powerful carbon-steel permanent magnets had become available in Europe; that heightened interest in their medical applications. These were intensively investigated by a highly respected Jesuit priest with the curious name of Maximilian Hell. He was also chief astronomer at the University of Vienna. Hell tried treating patients with steel magnets made into different shapes to correspond to the structures in the body that required healing, and recounted his numerous successes in a treatise published in 1762.

## The Doctor of Animal Magnetism

Hell's work with magnets had a profound influence on one of his younger academic colleagues, Franz Anton Mesmer. This is where we get the word "mesmerize." Despite his somewhat shady image today, he was a brilliant doctor.

Mesmer has been described as being quick-witted, with riveting eyes, and a flair for the theatrical. Well-trained in mathematics, medicine, and law, his doctoral thesis dealt with the effects of gravitational fields and cycles on human health. It proposed that an invisible magnetic energy permeated the universe, as well as all body fluids, and that the human body contained poles similar to a magnet. If these poles fell out of alignment with this universal flow, it could cause a variety of physical and emotional effects. He was obviously strongly swayed by Paracelsus, and equally convinced that magnets could cure such problems. In a 1775 report entitled *"On the Medicinal Uses of the Magnet,"* he vividly described how he had cured a patient with uncontrollable seizures and numerous other nervous system problems—by feeding her iron filings and applying Hell's specially shaped magnets:

> When my patient had another attack, I fixed two magnets of horseshoe-shaped type to her feet and a heart-shaped magnet to her breast. Suddenly she felt a burning sensation spreading from her feet through all her joints like a glowing coal . . . and likewise from both sides of the breast to the crown of the head . . . the pains gradually went away, she became insensitive to the magnets. The symptoms disappeared and she recovered from the seizure.

Mesmer subsequently experimented with placing the magnets on different parts of the patient's body, and she gradually improved. He was certain that the cure had resulted from his control of the flow of the "universal fluid" within her body, explaining in his memoirs that:

> Certain properties analogous to those of the magnet reveal themselves, especially in the human body. It is possible to distinguish different and opposite poles that may be changed, linked, destroyed or reinforced . . . This property of the human body, which makes it responsive to the influence of the heavenly bodies and to the reciprocal action of the bodies around it, made me, in view of the analogy with the magnet, call it animal magnetism *(magnetisomum animalem)*.

He distinguished this energy from that in iron and steel, which he referred to as "mineral" magnetism. He believed that he could "magnetize" wood, paper, water, or anything by virtue of his own animal magnetism, and that regular magnets simply served as conductors to facilitate the flow of "universal fluid" from him to the patient. Mesmer's animal magnetism produced some miraculous cures. One deaf patient had his hearing restored after Mesmer held his hands over the patient's ears. Others had instant relief of persistent chest or stomach spasms when he stroked these parts of their bodies. He traveled throughout Europe for the next two years, and his fame as a healer skyrocketed. In retrospect, it would appear that he had really discovered hypnosis, which we still refer to as mesmerism.

Mesmer's good friend, Mozart, gave him a plug in his popular comic opera *Cosi fan tutte*. Near the end of the first act, when two men pretend to take poison to test the loyalty of their fiancées, a maid speaks of seeking a marvelous doctor who cures people without a knife or a pill. She returns disguised as a doctor, and pulling out a giant magnet from under her costume, she touches the foreheads of the two faking invalids, then strokes their bodies with it, following which they magically recover. Her accompanying song is: "Here and there a touch of the magnet, the stone of Mesmer, who was born in Germany and became so famous in France."

Mesmer had indeed become one of the most famous and controversial figures of his time, especially in France. He was unable to accommodate the increasing number of patients who flocked to him, and sought ways to treat several simultaneously. His popularity and unorthodox treatment had not been received well by Vienna's conservative medical community, who viewed animal magnetism as a hoax, so Mesmer moved to Paris, where he established a salon of magnetic paraphernalia in the fashionable Place Vendôme. It was more show biz than medicine, but clients lapped it up.

Patients sat by wooden tubs known as baquets, which contained magnetized water and iron filings, and had projecting magnetized iron rods. The willing patients then poured magnetic water on affected parts of their bodies, or rubbed them against the rods, or simply grasped the rods. They also periodically joined hands to facilitate the flow of Mesmer's magnetic "universal fluid." "Assistant magnetizers" were on hand to provide help and instructions in these activities. All of this was conducted in a highly theatrical setting that included numerous mirrors, colored fabrics and lights, and dramatic piano music in the background. Everything was orchestrated and presided over by the maestro, who would intermittently appear with a long iron rod, using either this or his hands to perform healings. It was not unusual for a patient to faint or have a convulsive fit, and such a climax was viewed as a sign that healing would soon follow.

Mesmer's animal magnetism was hailed as a new force analogous to Newton's gravity, and Parisians waited in long lines to get into the salon. French physicians also considered him to be a fraud, but didn't know how to prove this to the hordes who wanted to be healed by Mesmer alone. Many of his most ardent followers were rich and famous, including Lafayette, the Revolutionary War hero, who wrote to his friend George Washington extolling the virtues of animal magnetism. But Mesmer's great public and financial success with royalty and aristocrats outraged many orthodox physicians of his day. The French Academy of Sciences finally convinced King Louis XVI to establish an unbiased royal commission in 1784, to determine whether Mesmer's treatment had any scientific validity. The three commissioners were Antoine Lavoisier, who first demonstrated the role of oxygen in respiration and fire, Benjamin Franklin from America, and Dr. J. I. Guillotin, whose name was later given to the very device that would behead the royalty and the aristocrats.

In an early version of the double-blind study, the commission members observed blindfolded patients who sat in front of powerful magnets, and asked them to describe their sensations, comparing these to their responses when fake objects were substituted without their knowledge. The panel concluded that magnetic healing was entirely due to the belief of the patient and the power of suggestion. Their opening statement pointed out in a rational fashion that "Animal magnetism might well exist without being useful, but it cannot be useful if it does not exist."

Mesmer countered by requesting that the commission select patients with various stubborn neuropsychiatric problems, and contrast the results of his treatment with those that the best conventional treatment could provide. The panel wisely refused, recognizing that many patients with such stress-related complaints might well improve, but not through any objective, biophysical energy that could be measured.

## Explorations into Electromagnetism

Scientists in the meantime were trying to unlock the mysteries of this force.

In 1820, a Danish physicist named Hans Christian Oersted was able to prove that an electric current flowing in a wire or coil produces its own magnetic field. He was in the midst of lecturing to a class of physics students when he made the discovery. By chance he had placed a wire carrying a current near the needle of a compass, and was startled to see the needle swing at right angles to the wire. Although Gilbert had shown 200 years previously that there was no link between lodestones and static electricity, this discovery showed a clear link between magnetism and electrical current.

In France, Andre-Marie Ampere quickly improved on the idea. A science teacher who was mostly self-educated, Ampere rose to become Inspector General of the French University system. He demonstrated the magnetic forces between electric conductors in mathematical terms: Ampere's law describes the magnetic field produced by a conductor carrying an electrical current.

During the 1820s, William Sturgeon of England and Joseph Henry of the United States independently developed electromagnets. By wrapping copper wire carrying a current of electricity around an iron bar, they magnetized it to the point where it could lift extremely heavy objects, eventually those weighing up to one ton. Today, electromagnets lift cars in junk yards and transport them to compactors.

Michael Faraday, the British chemist, was fascinated by science as a child and became one of the greatest experimental physicists. He gave magnetic force the name of magnetic field in 1845. His most important work was in connecting magnetism to electricity, interpreting the results of Oersted and Ampere. He showed that a moving magnet could produce an electric current, just as electricity in motion produces magnetism. Faraday created the first dynamo, which led to the development of the motor.

So the links in the chain of understanding continued to grow. Faraday's theories were extended by James Maxwell of Scotland (1831–1879). Maxwell was able to describe in mathematical terms the elegant similarities between electricity and magnetism, and that the movement of one created the other. His real breakthrough was showing that light is an electromagnetic phenomenon and predicting that there would be other energies in this category. His ideas were not accepted outside England until the German physicist Heinrich Hertz described electromagnetic waves traveling at the speed of light—today's radio waves.

Magnetism also fascinated Samuel Hahnemann, the founder of homeopathic medicine ("like cures like"). Homeopathic medicines are reduced, minuscule doses—so minuscule as to be almost nonexistent—of substances that produce the very symptoms the patient suffers. Hahnemann felt these substances would react with the life force of the body in the same way as they reacted to the lodestone. He also used the magnet in treatment.

Galvani and Volta, both of Italy, are names we instantly associate with electricity. Galvani could contract ("galvanize") muscles with electric current, and reasoned that the human body itself produced electricity. But he failed to account for the fact that it took two wires of different metals to produce the contractions. Volta went on to experiment and confirmed that it took two dissimilar metals to produce the electricity. Direct current (DC), continuously flowing electricity, was what they had discovered. Galvani's theories were not accepted, however, and he died neglected, while Volta invented the first battery—the first source of continuous electric current.

Magnetism attracted many other scientists who studied its properties in various ways. Among the names, you will recognize Louis Pasteur, Pierre and Marie Curie, and Albert Einstein.

# Magnets Come to America

Mesmer faded away, but magnetic therapy became extremely popular in the United States. This may have been spurred on by Benjamin Franklin's famous experiments with electricity. Elisha Perkins, a Connecticut physician, got a patent in 1795 for his "magnetic tractor" device that could "draw off the noxious electrical fluid that lay at the root of suffering," and made a fortune selling them for $25.00 each. A book entitled *The History and Philosophy of Animal Magnetism* was published by a "Practical Magnetizer" in Boston in 1843. Around the same time, Phineas Quimby, another follower of Mesmer, established his magnetic healing practice in Portland, Maine, which also used touch and the power of suggestion. One of the patients he cured was Mary Patterson, who became Mary Baker Eddy and founded Christian Science. Although originally a proponent of mesmerism, she came to believe that the only source of healing was prayer, and in later life, derided animal magnetism as being "malicious," and "the action of error in all its forms."

Mary Shelley's *Frankenstein,* published in 1818, stimulated interest in electricity as a source of life. Since limbs or other body parts would jump when electrical shocks were administered to animal and human cadavers, it was believed that electricity could bring the dead to life. There were various "reanimation" chairs, devices, and techniques—some of which may possibly have acted as defibrillators. One induction coil with sponge-tipped electrodes was successfully used to treat angina and arrhythmias in 1853 (fundamentally the same as the "paddles" so familiar to us from the hospital).

Around the same time, another coil was used to treat curvature of the spine, a treatment for scoliosis that has also been revived. After the Civil War, the use of permanent magnets soared, particularly in the newly industrialized farm belts in the West. Mail-order catalogues advertised magnetic boot soles for 18¢ a pair, and offered all sorts of genuine magnetic rings, belts, girdles, caps, and other apparel that could be used for everything from menstrual cramps to impotency and baldness. Magnetic salves and liniments were popular over-the-counter products, and were dispensed by traveling magnetic healers. Towards the end of the century, Daniel Palmer opened Palmer's School of Magnetic Cure in Davenport, Iowa, which emphasized the laying on of hands, massage, and manipulation that later became chiropractic therapy.

By the turn of the century, medical textbooks were devoting chapters to the use of magnetism and electricity for the treatment of neurological and emotional disorders. Electrotherapeutics was viewed as a legitimate subspecialty, much like the rapidly expanding fields of radiology and radium therapy. Electromagnetic therapy was used to treat anemia, convulsions, hysteria, insomnia, migraine, neuralgia, arthritis, fatigue, numerous emotional disorders, and any type of pain. There were numerous devices, with names like the "dynamiser" and "oscilloclast," based on theories that each organ and person were "tuned" to specific electromagnetic wavelengths that could rejuvenate them.

The king of magnetic healers was Dr. C. J. Thacher, whose Chicago's Magnetic Company promised "health without the use of medicine." His mail-order pamphlet explained that the energy responsible for life comes from the magnetic force of the sun, which is conducted through the rich iron content of the blood. Disease resulted when stressful lifestyles and environmental factors interfered with these healing forces.

However, "magnetism properly applied will cure every curable disease no matter what the cause." The most efficient way to expedite this ability of iron in the blood to transmit healing magnetic energy was by wearing magnetic clothing, and almost every conceivable garment was available. A complete costume, which promised "full and complete protection of all the vital organs of the body," contained 700 magnets. When interviewed in his State Street office, Thacher was wearing "a magnetic cap, a magnetic waistcoat, magnetic stocking liners, and magnetic insoles." As he explained to the reporter:

> My object is to spread the light, to rescue humanity. I can
> cure anything. I will compel the authorities to take notice of
> my methods . . . Let the authorities turn over ten cases to me.
> I'll put my magnetic shields on 'em and restore the harmo-
> nious vibrations of the brain, and everything will be well!
> Paralysis? An easy problem. Had five cases . . . Cured 'em
> right off. Winked. Spoke. Got up and walked. Paralysis? Pish!

Although Dr. Thacher was considered by federal authorities and the medical establishment as a quack, his magnetic insoles deserve another look. Last year a report in a prestigious medical journal described how magnets could relieve the symptoms of diabetic neuropathy, usually manifesting as complaints of pain, burning sensations, and/or loss of feeling in the lower extremities. There is no treatment for this condition, which tends to become progressively worse. The report described how such patients had relief of their pain following the continual use of magnetic insoles. At the end of four months, three out of four patients reported their pain had disappeared.

Furthermore, when they stopped wearing the magnets, symptoms returned. Dr. Thacher would be pleased: "Pain? Pish!" he might say.

Around his time, in the 1920s and afterward, all sorts of theories and contraptions made extravagant claims for cures, most of which were clearly worthless. The devices for the most part didn't live up to their claims. In addition, following World War II, the advent of antibiotics, cortisone, and other medical advances provided predictable scientific remedies for many conditions and magnetic therapy lost its allure. It was pushed back into the shadows of quackery.

Until now. Some of the wonder drugs have turned out to have a dark side, and alternative medicine has become a strong popular trend. As the medical paradigm shifts, doors open to different forms of healing, and magnetic therapy is being reevaluated—a new technology of design has come into being.

## A Short History of Medicine

| | |
|---|---|
| 2000 B.C. | Here, eat this root. |
| A.D. 1000 | That root is heathen. Here, say this prayer. |
| A.D 1850 | That prayer is superstition. Here, drink this potion. |
| A.D. 1940 | That potion is snake oil. Here, swallow this pill. |
| A.D. 1985 | That pill is ineffective. Here, take this antibiotic. |
| A.D. 2000 | That antibiotic is artificial. Here, eat this root. |

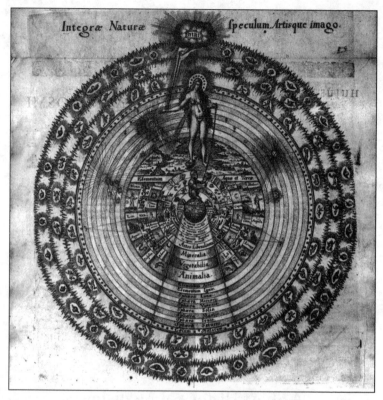

Robert Fludd's depiction of unity in the cosmos, extending from earth, through all the elements, the planets, and the stars. (Reproduced with permission from the Department of Printing and Graphic Arts, The Houghton Library, Harvard University.)

# Magnetism, Electricity, and Energy

*The true delight is in the finding out, rather than in the knowing.*

—Isaac Asimov

# Why Do Opposites Attract?

---

Magnets and magnetism have obviously fascinated mankind for thousands of years. Most of you may also recall your own wonder when you discovered magnets as a child. What was this weird force you couldn't see or feel? Why would a magnet stick to some things but not to others? And if you put the ends of two magnets close together, there might be a strong attraction; but if you switched one of them around, the reverse occurred. Why?

We later learned that all magnets had a north pole at one end, and a south pole at the other. Also, if a magnet was cut in half, or a sliver was sliced off, the remnants would still always have a north and south pole at either end. Scientists have tried for many years to isolate these two poles. However, no matter how small it is, anything magnetic always has a north and south pole, never one without the other. University of California physicists spent five years bombarding tens of billions of atomic nuclei with sophisticated techniques in a futile attempt to knock off one pole, and finally admitted complete defeat in 1997.

We sometimes describe a person as having a "magnetic personality," or say that "opposites attract." Is there some connection? Could people be like magnets in certain ways? When you finish this book, that won't sound as crazy as it may seem. Scientists have shown that all matter has some magnetic properties. And each of us does emit some strange sort of biomagnetic energy field that can be demonstrated with special imaging techniques. This also seems to vary with our state of physical and mental well-being, much like the ancient Chinese concept of *Qi*. Some suggest that the ability of a strong faith or determination to fight disease is related to having emotional or mental powers that can focus this force to promote healing. Renowned healers and *QiGong* masters seem to have more bio-magnetic energy and have learned how to harness it better. Some can even project it to influence others, even those several feet away. In chapter 10, we will show how this energy can be demonstrated in laboratory studies, which also reveal that it has the same effect as does a permanent magnet on chemical reactions responsible for energy formation in the body.

## Heading in the Right Direction

We also have tiny magnetic granules in our brains. Nobody knows why, but in many animals these particles seem to function like a compass. Millions of birds travel tremendous distances to reach their same winter and summer homes every year. They can do this without the aid of the sun or stars, when it is dark and cloudy. The most likely explanation is that the magnetite particles allow them to be guided by sensing the earth's magnetic field, which provides a sense of direction. The same may be true for whales and other sea life that have no visible cues to tell them where they are going. Magnetite can be found in bees, butterflies, and all kinds of creatures, where the particles may serve some similar navigational purpose. If you create an artificial magnetic field around the head of a homing pigeon, the bird's ability to reach its destination can be significantly impaired. Some people have a better sense of direction than others when they are blindfolded. This seems to diminish or disappear when they also wear a metallic covering that blocks the earth's magnetic field.

Exactly what is a magnet? A simple definition is "anything that attracts iron." If you sprinkle iron filings on a piece of paper that is placed on top of a magnet, the filings will promptly arrange themselves in a pattern that outlines the magnet's shape. As originally shown by William Faraday, who originated the concept of magnetic fields made up of flux lines, magnetic fields are strongest where the flux lines are closest together. The greatest concentration of iron filings are at the north and south poles of the magnet, since this is where the attractive force is greatest and the lines are closest. There are almost no iron filings around the middle of the magnet, where the force is weakest (see figure 2.1). The same can be shown with a bar magnet, or for that matter, several magnets.

People have been puzzled for centuries about what causes magnetism. The answer is that magnets consist of millions of minuscule units containing atoms that assemble in groups called domains. Each domain acts like a miniature magnet with a north and a south pole. When the domains become aligned in the same direction, their force combines to make a larger magnet with the same north and south poles. Iron has many domains just waiting to line up in some direction, so it is easy to magnetize. Because domains in plastic and rubber are scattered in a disorderly fashion, their magnetic fields tend to cancel each other out; therefore, no overall polarity results (see figure 2.2). When a piece of iron or steel is placed close enough to be affected by a magnet's field, it will become magnetized to the extent that its domains can be aligned in the same direction as that of the magnet. This effect is called residual or induced magnetism.

An iron nail can be readily magnetized, but its power fades away fairly quickly. Magnetizing a steel needle takes longer, although once this has been accomplished, the needle's magnetic properties are more persistent (see figure 2-3). Another way to demonstrate induced magnetism is to pick up a chain of

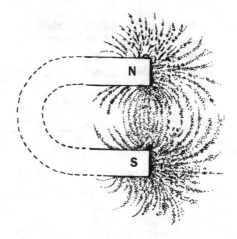

**Figure 2.1**

Note that iron filings gather primarily at the poles,
where the lines of magnetic flux are closest.

paper clips or pins with a magnet. The stronger the magnet,
the longer the chain will be. The clips closest to the magnet
will be the most powerful, and even when you subsequently
remove the magnet, some clips may retain enough residual
magnetism that they will continue to attract each other. Clips
farther away from the magnet that are separate will not show as
much of this tendency. If you drop a magnet on a hard surface, or hit it with a hammer, it may not remain as strong,
because some of the domains are knocked out of line.
Extreme heat will also cause a magnet to lose its strength.

## Putting Magnets on the Map,
## Literally and Figuratively

William Gilbert put magnets on the map not only figuratively,
but literally. He accurately explained why a compass needle

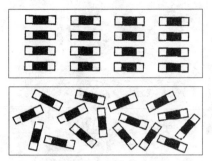

**Figure 2.2**

The upper section shows the orderly formation of domains in a magnetized metal. The lower section shows the haphazard arrangement of nonmagnetic substances such as wood or rubber.

pointed north, and also aimed down as it was taken closer to the North Pole. Many believe his 1600 book *De Magnete (About Magnets)* is the first real example of scientific writing because it illustrates such an objective, orderly, and comprehensive approach.

Magnets started out as a hobby for Gilbert, but soon became his obsession. He read everything he could get his hands on about the lodestone from Greek, Roman, Arabic, and East Indian sources, but apparently knew little about Oriental views. He quickly became confused by the contradictory opinions about how magnets should be used to promote health, much as some people are today. For example, Aristotle and Galen said magnets were "cold," while Hippocrates and leading Arabic physicians claimed they were "hot." This may require some explanation.

## A Little Humour Can Go a Long Way

At the time, Galen's theory of the four humours had dominated medicine for well over a thousand years. The ancient

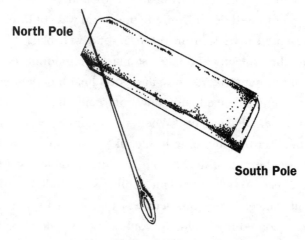

**North Pole**

**South Pole**

**Figure 2.3**

A needle can be magnetized by stroking it against one of the
magnet's poles and is said to have residual, or induced, magnetism.

Greeks believed that there were only four elements: fire, water,
air, and earth. These perpetual substances were considered
ageless, indestructible, and responsible for everything in the
world. Each had its own character, and although equally important, one would dominate the other on occasion. Something like the paper, scissors, rock game kids play with their
hands—scissors can cut paper, paper can cover rock, but a
rock can break scissors. So which is strongest?

Like everything else on earth, the human body was composed of the four elements, which later came to be associated
with one of the four "humours" that Galen taught were responsible for regulating physical and mental health. There was
blood, choler (yellow bile), melancholy (black bile), and
phlegm. Each was associated with different organs, and each
possessed two of the four primary qualities: hot, cold, wet, and

dry. Thus, blood came from the heart and was hot and wet; phlegm diffused down from the brain and was cold; yellow bile represented dryness from the liver; and wet, black bile came from the spleen and the stomach. Humours circulated through the mind and body, and good health depended upon their being balanced, not only internally, but with external environmental elements. When the humours were knocked out of kilter by something inside, like bad thoughts, or by outside weather conditions, such as "unfavorable" winds, one would become sick. What kind of illness depended on the type of imbalance. If the problem was too much heat, then one needed something "cold" to counteract the "hot," or to find some other way to restore balance. That's why bloodletting, leeches, and "cupping" were popular treatments for so long, and still are in some parts of the world.

The Greeks believed that these humours also determined one's "temperament" or "complexion" because, like the Chinese, they made no distinction between mind and body. An excess of one humour could make a person sanguine (Latin for blood), melancholy, choleric (bilious, easily provoked, revengeful), or phlegmatic (sluggish, indifferent). Some of these words have lost their significance, but we still describe individuals as being "ill-humored," "hot-" and "cold-blooded," or "chilly" and as "venting their spleen" or having a "jaundiced" view.

If you want to appease someone, you "humor" them. Many people all over the world also remain convinced that they can get sick when certain regional winds prevail, when there are frequent changes in the weather, or when they catch a chill from being cold. Like *Qi*, these humours were constantly exchanging information with the external environment. It's important to emphasize how ingrained these notions were, and that "humour" was the Greek word for fluid. This is the reason why everyone from Gilbert to Benjamin Franklin were so sure that electricity was some sort of liquid.

Plato had described magnets as being "divine," and Aristotle believed that, in addition to attracting iron, they possessed numerous other powers that were "all undiscovered." Gilbert, who was even more in awe, wrote:

A lodestone is a wonderful thing in many experiments and like a living thing. And one of its remarkable virtues is that which the ancients considered to be a living soul in the sky, in the globes, and in the stars, in the sun and in the moon.

While this was pure speculation, science seems to be showing us more and more that Gilbert was right. Magnetic forces are involved in everything in the universe, from the orbits of planetary bodies and their satellites, to the spin of electrons in atoms, and perhaps to the communication that takes place between everything.

## Peter the Pilgrim
## and How to Catch an Adulteress

Gilbert was fascinated by Peter Peregrinus. In 1269, the city of Lucera in Italy was under siege by order of the Pope because its citizens had strayed from the faith. One of those helping in this campaign was Pierre de Maricourt, an engineer who became Peter Peregrinus. Peregrinus, which means pilgrim, was a title the Pope bestowed from time to time to reward those doing "God's work." Peregrinus was trying to see whether he could make a perpetual motion machine with lodestones he carved into the shape of a sphere. He sent a lengthy letter to a friend describing how different parts of a lodestone acted on a sliver of iron, how a lodestone that he floated tended to line up in a north-south direction and would return to that position whenever he tried to make it point otherwise. If he floated two lodestones so that their ends were close, they would try to come together, and, when he turned one to face in the opposite direction, the reverse would happen. Peregrinus, who may have been the first to recognize that all magnets had a north and a south end, coined the term "polus" to refer to this; we still call the ends poles. He also showed how a lodestone could be used to make a piece of iron magnetic. He conducted all these experiments while camped outside the city, trying to figure out a way to break down its walls.

In addition to reading everything he was able to get his hands on, Gilbert collected information about what magnets could do and how they worked from any source. He found no lack of old wives' tales and superstition. Magnets could keep evil spirits away and thus prevent things like spasms and gout which they might inflict. Wearing garlic cloves and diamonds was thought to be another way to keep evil spirits away, because they had strange powers over magnets. If a lodestone "be anointed with garlic" or a diamond is close by, "it does not attract iron." Ground-up lodestones helped spleen and liver problems, and moved sluggish bowels because of their laxative effect, which promoted "due evacuations; for which reason it restores young girls when pallid, sickly, and lacking color, to health and beauty." There's little doubt that iron can cure anemia in young girls (who often have a deficiency due to heavy periods and poor nutrition), but not because it relieves constipation. This is another example demonstrating that theories don't have to be correct; only facts do. Such applies to magnets today. Many current theories about why magnets work are incorrect. What is important are the facts, and the fact is that they do work, even if we don't completely understand why or how.

Another notion was that if one put a lodestone under the head of a woman while she was sleeping, it would force her to get out of bed if she had committed adultery. It could remove a sorcerer's spell, improve marriages, and "make one acceptable and in favor with princes." Some viewed it as the long-sought-after elixir of life, while "others relate that lodestone perturbs the mind and makes folk melancholic and mostly kills." Lodestones could apparently do anything. Gilbert was amazed at all this confusion and misinformation about his beloved magnets. As far as he was concerned, the application of a lodestone for all sorts of headaches "no more cures them (as some say) than would an iron helmet or a steel cap." He was determined to separate fact from fancy by personally subjecting every theory to scientific scrutiny. He did debunk most of them, but failed to explain how magnets identified unfaithful wives.

Peregrinus wondered how these myths originated, and found one source providing information. At around the same time Peter Peregrinus was camped out in Italy, a man named Bartholomew wrote an encyclopedia intended to provide authoritative information on everything that was known. Concerning magnets, he stated:

This kind of stone restores husbands to wives and increases elegance in charm and speech. Moreover, along with honey, it cures dropsy, spleen, fox mange and burn. . . . When placed on the head of a chaste woman, it causes its poisons to surround her immediately, but if she is an adulteress she will immediately remove herself from bed for fear of an apparition.

As such myths were passed down from one generation to another, they were often exaggerated, as are stories concerning how big a fish someone caught. Bartholomew also wrote that "there are mountains of such stones and they attract and dissolve ships of iron," which must have terrified thirteenth-century seamen. That story keeps resurfacing, and was in fact the subject of a movie several years ago, in which magnetic fields made a battleship disappear.

## East Is East and West Is West, But North and South Always Try to Meet

William Gilbert was the first to recognize that the earth itself was a huge magnet with a north and south pole, which deviated from the geographic poles. He also explained why a compass needle would be increasingly deflected downward as ships got closer to the North or South Pole. He discovered that iron rods in buildings or windows whose ends had been pointing north and south for 20 years or more had become weakly magnetized. This didn't happen when the alignment was east-west. In Gilbert's day, magnets were made by hammering a

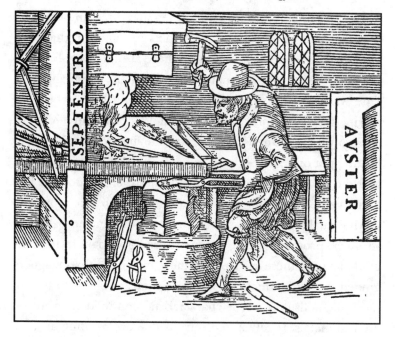

**Figure 2.4**

In the sketch above from *De Magnete, Septentrio* is an early English word that refers to the north, and *Auster* means southerly.

lodestone into a molten iron bar with ends pointed to the north and south poles to take advantage of the earth's magnetic field (see figure 2.4).

## How Are Modern Magnets Made?

Gilbert also noted that when a piece of iron had been struck by lightning, it could become magnetized. Magnets are now made by passing a strong surge of DC electricity through a bar containing iron; this has the same effect as lightning because it also causes domains to line up in the same direction. Magnets that are used to treat aches and pains are mass-produced in huge batches to reduce costs, and there are relatively few suppliers. Most magnet companies buy from the same supplier. One who wishes to buy magnets may ask, why not buy the cheapest if two brands come from the identical source? There are two reasons. One is that not just the magnet itself, but the coating put on it, and other characteristics related to flexibility and durability of the material being used, are important factors. In addition, different grades, ranging from 1–5, represent varying quality and consistency; higher ratings mean better or stronger products. Most magnets used for pain relief are graded 4 or 5; these are typically more expensive than magnets graded 1, 2, or 3, which will not do the job as well.

Magnetism is not a characteristic confined to iron, or even to metals. It refers to electrons that are orbiting around their atoms. Electrons have a property called spin, which makes them act like miniature magnets with a north and south pole. If you force a lot of neighboring electrons in anything to spin so that their poles are aligned in the same direction, you can make it magnetic. Iron is very easy to magnetize because it has lots of surplus electrons hanging around that will readily line up any way you want them to. But some nonmetallic substances also have enough spare electrons to do this without much difficulty. Scientists have now been able to make almost anything into a magnet that will stick to a refrigerator door, including paper, as will be explained in chapter 10.

The magnets in current use are much more powerful because of their composition. We have come a long way from lodestones, which are made magnetic by bacteria that need iron in their diet, which they convert into magnetite. Iron was supplanted in the early 1700s by carbon-steel magnets that were more powerful and longer-lasting. Around 100 years ago, advances in steel-making led to stronger alloy magnets containing tungsten, cobalt, chromium, or molybdenum. These were surpassed, in the 1930s, by iron-based products containing aluminum, nickel, and cobalt (called alnico magnets). A decade or two later, magnets containing barium and strontium became available; although not as powerful, these were much cheaper to use for manufacturing motors and speakers. In 1970, the first rare earth magnets made of cobalt and samarium were introduced; these were significantly superior. But cobalt could only be obtained from foreign sources and became prohibitively expensive for mass commercial use. Therefore, in 1983, rare earth magnets composed of iron, boron, and neodymium, dubbed "neo" magnets, began to be manufactured. They are more permanent, with almost no detectable loss of strength over ten years or more.

What is it that makes a magnet more powerful? To comprehend this, it is necessary to consider complex qualities like saturation magnetization, coercivity, and maximum energy, characteristics that are much too technical to try to explain here. The important thing to understand is that adding these rare earth or trace metals to iron makes it possible to produce magnets that are much smaller but more powerful than previous ones several times their size. Magnets were formerly made in the shape of a bent horseshoe, so that the pulling power of both poles could be used to lift something. A single pole of a modern neodymium magnet is so powerful that this is no longer necessary. In addition, because these new magnets don't corrode like iron, they last longer. Advances in the design and composition of magnets have hinged on economic advantages in enormous mass markets for electronic devices such as computer hard disks and audio and video recording tapes. While this also provides definite advantages for magnets used to treat patients, factors other than those that concern manufacturers of electronic devices may influence how magnets work in the body.

Modern magnets are more powerful than most people think. After the Iron Curtain dropped, a prime-time television show was devoted to demonstrating the power Russian psychics had to attract or move objects without touching them. Many of the objects contained iron or steel, and it seemed likely that the "psychic powers" depended on carefully concealed magnets. Magnetic field strength falls off very quickly as you move away from its source. Magnetic strength is easily calculated, since it varies with the square of the distance. If mattress magnets are four inches away from your body, then their strength is only $\frac{1}{16}$th of their gauss rating (a gauss is a unit that tells the strength of the magnetic field).

Therefore, you would need an awful lot of magnets to experience any effect, or they would have to be very powerful. And they are. A modern magnet small enough to be hidden under a fingernail can make a compass needle swing around from a considerable distance.

But it is doubtful that even these magnets can live up to the claims made for some commercial applications. In *Driving Force,* a very informative and entertaining book which is highly recommended (Harvard University Press, 1996), James Livingston gives several examples. One is a company that offers Magnalawn 200, which is described as "a magnetohydrodynamic fertilizer utilizing chemical-free natural magnetic energy." It contains powerful magnets in a device that you can attach to your garden hose that will "neutralize the harmful chemicals found in water, reduce water consumption up to 40%, and promote healthier soil and growth conditions." Other magnetic products promise to soften tap water, sharpen razor blades, and prevent corrosive damage to metallic pipes. A real winner is a $45 doughnut-shaped magnet through which you can pour wine. Allegedly, pouring the wine over the north pole will give you a "rich and tangy taste," while the south provides a "smooth and sweet" flavor. The FDA monitors health claims, but how is truth in advertising enforced? If hype about magnets gives them a bad name, it surely will spill over into their medical applications.

# How Did Electricity Get into the Act?

What has magnetism to do with electricity, and what's the difference between a magnet and an electromagnet? Electricity, as we know it, is a very new kid on the block compared to magnetism. Although lightning has been around since the earth was created, nobody knew what it was, or what caused it. The ancient Greeks thought they were thunderbolts from Zeus, and other cultures also viewed them as a sign that some deity was angry. At times, lightning was also perceived as a divine source of energy that could bring life. We see this in Michelangelo's depiction of God's finger giving the spark of life to Adam on the ceiling of the Sistine Chapel. We also find it in the story of Dr. Frankenstein, who harnessed the power of lightning to create his monster. It took Benjamin Franklin to finally figure out that lightning was a form of electricity, but the story really begins in Italy, with a frog.

Amber has long been used to make necklaces and bracelets, and the attractive force that results when you rub it has been known for centuries. Kids create it by rubbing a comb or a plastic pen on their sleeve so it will pick up little pieces of paper. Although Gilbert had shown that rubbing glass and other things could also make them attract objects, he named this force electricity, after the Greek word for amber. Since he knew from his experience with magnets that two things had to be opposite to be attracted to each other, he referred to these two different fluid forces as resinous and vitreous electricity. Electricity was caused by removal of a fluid, or "humour," which then left an "effluvium," or atmosphere, around the object. The language is quaint, but, if you change "humour" to "charge" and "effluvium" to "electric field," his description is pretty close to our current concept.

Magnets could only attract iron, but what we now call static electricity could attract feathers and your hair. The power was not as strong as magnetism. If you put a piece of parchment in the way, rubbed amber couldn't pick up anything; parchment had no effect on a magnet's pull. However, if you produced lots of friction, it was possible to generate a spark of electricity you could see and feel; this phenomenon didn't happen with magnets. You couldn't make a magnet stronger by doing anything. Many people tried making friction wheels they could turn fast enough to cause a spark of static electricity. Some could give you a mild shock, such as the kind you get after walking over a carpet and putting a key in a lock on a cold, dry day. Others would produce a twitch, and were used in anatomy laboratories to study how different muscles reacted.

In the early 1700s, Peter van Musschenbrock at the University of Leyden was trying to see if he could make sparks he was generating travel through a wire coming out of a glass jar an assistant held; it worked. After the experiment was over and the wheel had stopped, van Musschenbrock took the glass jar back, and happened to touch the wire coming out of its neck. He got the shock of his life, literally and figuratively. "Suddenly I received in my right hand a shock of such violence, that my whole body was shaken as by a lightning stroke. The arm and the body were affected in a manner more terrible than I can express. In a word, I believed that I was done for." Actually, he had discovered a way to store electricity. He subsequently constructed a jar with a lining of tinfoil on the inside and on the outside. He filled it with electricity from the friction machine, and found that, if he was careful, he could carry it around the laboratory to use when he needed electricity without having to crank up the generator each time. This so-called Leyden jar became very popular as an investigative tool in laboratories all over Europe. Modern storage devices that work on the same principle are called capacitors.

# The Italian Connection

Luigi Galvani, Professor of Anatomy at the University of Bologna, had been studying the anatomy of frog legs, and had an electrical generator in his laboratory. In 1780, one of his assistants, a relative named Giovanni Aldini, was working on a frog leg attached to the spinal cord dissection. He was shocked (but not with electricity) when the leg contracted as his scalpel touched the spinal column or a nerve. Someone else thought they had seen a spark from the nearby charged generator at the same time. Galvani repeated the experiment himself several times, with identical results. However, the reaction seemed to be much stronger when the generating machine was being cranked up. Also, when he was sure to hold the scalpel only by its bone handle so that he didn't touch any of its metal, nothing happened. A leg placed inside a glass container could contract by itself when it was adjacent to a generator that was being turned. Galvani reasoned that the electricity was surely the cause of these contractions. However, because of Galen's influence, he didn't think of electricity the way we do. He believed the effect had to be due to the transfer of some special humour or fluid, which he called "animal electricity."

In another experiment, Galvani found that he could make a dead frog dance without the generator, by holding it with a brass hook in one hand, and lowering it until its feet rested on a silver box. When he touched the box with a piece of metal held in his other hand, there was a pronounced twitch. If his assistant touched the box with the same piece of metal or anything else, nothing happened. However, if he held Galvani's hand and then touched the metal box, the dead frog jumped again. How could this happen if there was no source of electricity? The most logical explanation was that the animal humour was able to flow once the circuit was completed. He concluded that muscles acted like little Leyden jars that stored electricity until the circuit was completed.

Unfortunately, he never pursued this since he was involved in experiments with his electrostatic generator. He found that when he hung several frogs' legs from a wire surrounding the machine and cranked it up, "he was rewarded by the sight of all the legs jumping together." Galvani went bonkers. He hooked up frog legs to each of the door hinges in his house and created a circuit so he could make them all jump simultaneously. His wife and Aldini also got the bug when they found they could make dead chickens and sheep twitch, and ears wiggle and eyes blink on their amputated heads. Aldini decided to go on tour, and traveled all over Europe showing how he could make the legs of dead animals move and kick. On one occasion, the corpse of a murderer was made available to him by the President of the London College of Surgeons an hour after execution. Aldini demonstrated how he could made its extremities move as if the dead man were walking or lifting something.

Meanwhile, back at the Galvani ranch, which was getting to look more like a slaughterhouse with all the carcasses of dead animals and legless frogs lying around, Galvani and his wife were still plugging, or rather dissecting, away. During a thunderstorm, Galvani hung an iron rod in the air so that it did not touch the ground, attaching the spinal cord–frog legs dissection at the bottom, to which a wire was connected that went down into a well. Sounds like a Rube Goldberg contraption, but sure enough, whenever there was a flash of lightning, the legs immediately twitched, and before he could hear any thunder—Eureka!

Galvani had discovered that lightning was the same kind of electricity that he could produce with his generator. This really turned him on. The Galvanis had a hanging garden, and to make it a little more attractive (or at least more exciting), he would stick brass hooks in the spinal cords of his frog-leg preparations, and suspend them from the iron railing around the garden, so that he and his assistants could watch them all jump together whenever there was lightning. It's not clear whether he invited the neighbors over to see the show, or how often it happened.

One day, he noted that even though his specimens weren't attached to the iron rod he used to attract lightning, they still often twitched during a thunderstorm. What made it more confusing, it sometimes happened on sunny days when everything was quiet. That meant that the air contained some kind of electricity other than lightning that you couldn't see, hear, or feel. But what could it be? This became very frustrating to Galvani, and since these strange occurrences were rare, he had to keep getting fresh specimens. (Some estimate that

Galvani may have single-handedly destroyed half the frog population in Italy!) He finally gave up—not because he ran out of frogs, or in frustration, but rather because of his conviction that he had probably been imagining things because of wishful thinking. (That's not hard to believe if you consider how much time he, Mrs. Galvani, or somebody else had to sit around doing nothing but watch frog legs dangle in the air and try to detect the slightest twitch.) As he wrote, "In experimenting, it is easy to be deceived . . . and to think that we have seen and detected things which we wish to see and detect."

You have to feel sorry for Galvani. He worked so hard that he thought he was going nuts. And he was so close to grabbing the brass ring on the merry-go-round he had created. He is still remembered through such words as galvanize, galvanometer, and galvanic current, but he could have done much better. It was another Italian contemporary, Alessandro Volta, who put the pieces together, and whose name is much more familiar. But before we get to him, we have to cross the Atlantic and go back in time to Benjamin Franklin. You may remember that he was one of the three-man tribunal convened by the Royal French Academy of Science at the request of the king to investigate Mesmer. While Franklin had always been popular in France, where he had served as U.S. ambassador, he had been selected to cross-examine Mesmer because of a famous experiment he had performed thirty-two years previously.

## Go Fly a Kite

In 1747, Franklin proposed that all materials possess a single kind of electrical fluid that could neither be created nor destroyed. Amber would continue to attract things whenever it was rubbed, no matter what you did to it, or how many times you had rubbed it previously. When you rubbed something, it simply transferred some of the fluid from one object to another. Most people thought that it was the friction that created the electricity. They didn't recognize that when amber was rubbed with silk to make it attract things, an equal amount of opposite electricity or charge remained on the silk. Franklin thought this power was strong enough to penetrate things and that the rubbing transferred this electrical fluid from one thing to another. He renamed Gilbert's "vitreous fluid" positive electricity, and "resinous" became negative. Franklin assumed the direction of the electrical flow or current should be from positive to negative, since it was believed that a magnetic field flowed from the north, or positive pole, to the south. We still use positive and negative to describe electrical charges, even though we know it isn't a fluid, and we also know that an electrical current flows from negative to positive.

You may remember that Leyden jars used to store electricity could be discharged by touching the inner and outer foil layers simultaneously, and that doing so would give one a pretty good shock. And if you used a metal conductor to complete the circuit, there would be a bright spark. Franklin thought that lightning was a similar kind of electricity and tried to think of some way this could be convincingly demonstrated. How he had time to fool around with this is baffling. After all, he was responsible for the Franklin stove, bifocals, the U.S. Post Office, the Library System, *Saturday Evening Post, Poor Richard's Almanac,* getting England to sign a treaty with France when nobody else could, and who knows what else! Anyway, between all this, he managed to prove his theory.

In 1752, during a thunderstorm, he flew a kite with a metal tip. The kite was attached to a wet hemp line (which could conduct electricity), at the end of which he attached a metal key. Wrapped around the key was a thin silk rope, which he held. The metal tip would attract any electricity in the air, which would then travel down the wet hemp to the key, but not to his hand, since the silk would not conduct electricity. The experiment was a huge success; he found that whenever he moved his knuckles near the key, he could draw sparks from it. It was also a very dangerous experiment; the next two people who tried it were killed.

## Born with a Silver Spoon in His Mouth, and He Used It

Back to Alessandro Volta, who was born into an aristocratic family, but was down-to-earth—very friendly, good-natured, and outgoing. Volta became fascinated with electricity as a child, and had learned all he could about it in school. Born five years before Franklin flew his kite, Volta developed his own theory about electricity by the time he was only eighteen. He proposed that when you rubbed silk with a glass, or even your hand, what we call static electricity also came from some sort of force that was inside the object being rubbed. Normally, the attraction between the things that this internal electrical fluid was composed of was balanced, but when you disturbed it by vigorous rubbing, they got displaced. As a result, some charges were now free to attract other things. So while

Franklin proposed that there was one electrical fluid, Volta had a two-fluid theory, or something along those lines.

He was a Professor at the University of Pavia in 1791 when he heard of Galvani's theory that some sort of animal electrical fluid stored in muscle was released when his assistant held his hand to complete the circuit (and no other source of electricity was present). Volta admired Galvani's frog experiments, but thought the notion that muscles stored electricity like little Leyden jars was ridiculous. He repeated the experiment and confirmed what Galvani had found, but instead of an electrostatic generator, he used the electricity stored in a Leyden jar. He also discovered he could make a headless grasshopper sing by stimulating its vocal cords with electricity. Since he was a physicist, not a doctor, he didn't like to work with dead animals, and instead used live frogs in his experiments. He found he could make them twitch not only with the stored electricity in his jar, but also when they were touched by a circuit consisting of two different metals. How could that be explained?

One possibility was that the animal had some sort of electrical fluid whose normal flow was disturbed when it was attached to an external circuit, and this caused the twitching. He experimented on himself by putting some tin on the tip of his tongue and letting it come in contact with a silver spoon that was touching the back of his mouth. He immediately noted an unpleasant taste. People with silver fillings in their teeth sometimes experience this when they accidentally touch one with a spoon made of different metal. So the idea that stored electricity was what made muscles twitch was not the only explanation. Contact with certain metals that were different, he discovered, could somehow generate electricity.

So far, almost everyone we've talked about sooner or later became obsessed with magnetism or electricity. Perhaps obsession is an occupational hazard that's contagious. In any event, Volta was not immune; like Galvani, he went off on an experimental spree. (We know about Mrs. Galvani, who caught the bug herself, but what about the wives of the others? Were they "electromagnetic widows"?) What Volta essentially found after numerous investigations was that the most important thing for demonstrating the effects of different metals was water. You needed something moist at the interface to generate electricity between two different metals. It was the moisture that conducted the electricity; frog tissue itself wasn't important. And distilled water wouldn't work because it didn't conduct electricity. It was the tiny ions with different charges that we'll speak about later that were important, just as we believe they are important in understanding why magnets work as a medical treatment.

# When Things Pile Up,
# It Can Be Shocking

Volta now turned to seeing how much electricity he could make by connecting different metals with a moist conductor. The only way he could determine the strength of the current, which he called electromotive force, was by periodically testing it, with his tongue, or by seeing how strong a shock it would give him. He could have found out by seeing how much it deflected the needle of a compass, but that was not discovered until sometime later. His voltaic cell was made up of alternating layers of silver and zinc or copper and zinc separated by moist cardboard. You could pile them up on top of each other to get an added effect, which is why they are often referred to as voltaic piles. Some piles that were eight feet high could give a real jolt.

Alessandro Volta had invented the first battery. By now it was 1800 and he was fifty-five years old and had somehow found time to sire three sons since his marriage at age forty-nine. His wife must have said "That's enough with the work," so he gave up his research to spend more time with his family, and never tried to make money from his invention. Because of the battery's ability to make electricity so readily and cheaply, voltaic cells popped up everywhere. They were used to extract metals from ores. Currents from cells placed in water produced gas bubbles of hydrogen and oxygen, and different gases could be formed depending on what was in the water. Sir Humphrey Davy became famous for such studies. He was the first person to get high on nitrous oxide, or laughing gas, which later became a popular anesthetic. Davy discovered sodium and potassium and eventually identified forty-seven new elements. Volta made all this possible, but some credit should go to Galvani, and to the thousands of Italian frogs who literally "croaked" to advance the cause of science.

# Marrying Magnetism and Electricity

Most individuals who subsequently contributed to our present understanding of electricity were discussed in the previous chapter. But a few, especially Michael Faraday, require further explanation. Faraday developed the concept of a magnetic field with lines of force, or flux as he called them. He sketched how these fields looked when more than one magnet was placed under a piece of paper covered with iron filings. But these lines were only in Faraday's mind since, when he tapped the paper a few times, the filings quickly gravitated to either pole of the magnet, depending on which was closer. His great insight was recognizing that these lines of force extended out from the magnet to create a field, and that the energy was in the field, not in the magnet. Moreover, it did not flow like electricity from one pole to another since they had no beginning or end but were continuous. Some form of electricity had to be involved. What was the connection?

Meanwhile, in Denmark, Hans Christian Oersted had also been convinced that there was some link between electricity and magnetism. He had heard that when lightning struck a ship, it sometimes reversed the polarity of the compass needle. That meant it had to be remagnetized by rubbing it with another magnet. He also felt that if an electric current produced a magnetic field, it would probably best be demonstrated by using a very thin wire. He had already shown that if he passed a current through a wire, he could cause it to get hot or even incandescent if the charge was very great or the wire extremely thin. Since heat and light radiated out into space from the wire, magnetism might also.

Oersted planned to perform such an experiment for his students during the winter of 1820, but didn't have time to try it before his lecture on electricity. However, during his presentation, he noticed that when he ran a current through a wire, the needle of a compass lying near it seemed to move slightly.

Nobody made much of the occurrence, and it was several months before he tried the experiment again. Now there was no doubt about the effect; and when he used a thicker wire, the effect was much stronger. More importantly, he could not block the response by putting something between the wire and the compass. Oersted had discovered that an electric current could produce a magnetic field.

Faraday was excited about Oersted's discovery, since he reasoned that the reverse should also be true. He set out to prove it with a series of ingenious experiments. He had also heard that Joseph Henry in the U.S. had built a powerful electromagnet by winding a coil of wire around an iron bar, and that when he reversed the current, the polarity of the magnet instantly changed.

In the 1831 experiment, a voltaic cell produced a current that could be sent through a coil of insulated wire wrapped around the left half of an iron ring. A separate coil of insulated wire was wound around the right half of the ring, and its ends were joined over a compass. When the switch was closed so the current flowed into the first coil, a magnetic field was generated in the iron ring. That field then passed into the second coil and generated a brief current that caused the compass needle to move. He was also surprised to note that the needle moved in the opposite direction when he turned the current off. Faraday had discovered and proved magnetic induction. (Most of the historical information and quotes are adapted from *Hidden Attraction* by Garrit Verschuur, which is a highly recommended source of information.)

Faraday then showed that he could produce a steady current by moving a magnet in and out of a wire coil whose ends were joined over a magnet. The current occurred only while the magnet was in motion. This was the reverse of the electro-magnet.

Finally, in a "Rube Goldberg" device, Faraday suspended two magnets alongside wires fixed in bowls of mercury. (Mercury is a metal that conducts electricity and is liquid at room temperature.) When the current flowed through the wire, the magnet rotated around it. At the same time, the other wire would rotate around the other magnet. This demonstrated that electricity could have physical effects other than moving a compass needle. Faraday soon discovered the laws determining the production of electric currents by magnets, one of which was that the magnitude of the current was dependent upon the number of lines of force that were being intersected. He immediately recognized that he could produce a continuous current by rotating a copper disk between the poles of a powerful magnet and taking leads off the disk's rim and center. The outside of the disk would cut more lines than would the inside, and there would thus be a continuous current produced in the circuit linking the rim to the center. This was the first dynamo, which led to the development of the electric motor. By that time, it was obvious that you only had to reverse things and feed the current to the disk to make it rotate. The demand for magnets obviously skyrocketed when electricity became a household item, automobiles began to be built, and electric household and other appliances replaced mechanical ones.

## Faraday's Humourless Legacy

The burning question was whether the electric "fluid" apparently released by electric eels and torpedo fish, by a static electricity generator or by a voltaic battery, and by his new electromagnetic device were all the same, or were different fluids following different laws? Faraday was pretty sure that they were not fluids at all, but rather manifestations of the same force, but how could he prove it? He began a lengthy series of studies in 1832, designed to prove that all electricities had precisely the same properties and caused precisely the same effects. The key turned out to be electrochemical decomposition. Voltaic and electromagnetic electricity posed no problems, but static electricity did. He eventually satisfied himself and the rest of the world that he was correct, and that electricity was not a fluid, at least not in the sense of being a liquid, or "humour" (by this time, Galen was pretty much passé anyway).

Faraday's studies and research led him to a new theory of electrochemistry, mathematical formulae, and philosophy that later had profound influence on appreciating the existence of a much wider range of electromagnetic energies. While the theory is too complex to go into here, it had important implications for understanding why magnets work and why adding different rare elements confer different properties, depending on their atomic weights. When electric charges are transmitted from one place to another, the flow of electricity is said to be a current. For many years, electricity was actually thought to be a fluid (like water) that flowed through conductors (such as metal wires) and remained trapped in insulators like water in a reservoir.

What is the difference between an "electric field" and a "magnetic field"? Actually, both are usually all around us, since they are present wherever there is electricity. Both an electric and electromagnetic field (EMF) exist around power lines, appliances, light fixtures, and electric wiring; but electromagnetic fields are generated only when current is flowing through a wire. Electric fields are produced by the voltage on a wire. Most people don't realize that if you plug in a lamp or an appliance, even though it is not turned on, it will produce an electric field. When the light is lit or the appliance is running, both an electric and electromagnetic field will be present. It is the electromagnetic field from high power lines and electrical appliances that have caused the current cancer controversy, discussed in chapter 7. However, it is important to recognize that the term "magnetic" field is commonly used as a synonym for "electromagnetic" field, which is a field that is always moving. As Faraday demonstrated, a permanent magnetic field is stationary or still, unless you are moving the magnet. Permanent magnets are completely safe, and are not involved in this controversy.

As indicated above and in the previous chapter, Faraday provided much of the theoretical foundation for James Clerk Maxwell's 1863 unification of electric and magnetic phenomena by mathematical equations. These predicted the existence of electromagnetic waves, which twenty-three years later were verified by Heinrich Hertz, who was able to confirm their presence. Their use in long-distance communication—"radio"—followed within two decades. Subsequently, the entire electromagnetic spectrum emerged, including x-rays, gamma rays, ultraviolet, infrared, and all forms of light, radar, television, and so on—all of which travel through space at exactly the same speed, just as Maxwell had predicted. Maxwell's equations are still being used by NASA and others to reach solar system destinations. Astronomical investigations of the farthest reaches of outer space depend on our ability to identify and interpret electromagnetic waves. These studies also confirm that the influence of magnetism is present throughout the entire universe.

The electron was discovered by Joseph Thomson only one hundred years ago; he demonstrated how a magnet could bend a beam of light in a cathode tube. However, none of this would have been possible had no one wondered why a lodestone made iron filings jump up and cling to it, or been curious why a compass needle pointed north-south, or determined to learn how to make a dead frog's leg twitch.

# CHAPTER 3

# The Many Faces
# of Pain

- Painkillers
- Acupuncture
- Osteopuncture
- The Electro Side: TENS, NET, and LEET
- Auricular Medicine for Pain
- A Glance at Pain Research Today

*All the happiness mankind can gain*
*Is not in pleasure, but in rest from pain.*

—John Dryden

**A**ll humans have felt it; we all know what it is. It's a message—an unwelcome electrochemical message—running along nerve fibers to the brain and back again. It ranges from a mild, tolerable ache to a piercing burn, all the way up to an onslaught so overwhelming that awareness closes down and you lose consciousness. But even in its mildest form, pain is a warning signal that something is wrong. And, to add insult to injury, pain is also subjective—only the person who is suffering can really know how much it hurts.

Putting aside the subjective, facing only the actual, here's how pain works. The first signaling step occurs in the surface of nerve endings, which react to tissue damage by secreting a peptide known as substance P (P standing for pain). This substance activates nerve fibers that conduct pain messages through the central nervous system in nano-seconds.

Some pain sensations may be intercepted in the spinal cord, sidetracked to the thalamus before going on to the cerebral cortex. About the size of a walnut, the thalamus is a kind of Pain Central, receiving and relaying the warning-signal messages. It is believed to be more primitive, in the evolutionary sense, than the cerebral cortex, the "higher" brain. Interestingly, both these parts of the brain have been found to have "maps" of the body, so that impulses from a certain site on the "map" will go to that specific related site in the body.

"Phantom pain" sometimes occurs in the limbs of amputees, and is very resistant to control. In a few of these patients, continuous electrical stimulation of the thalamus has provided some relief. Current research is trying to find a way to block "spontaneous activity" in the thalamus that is thought to cause phantom sensations. In the past it was demonstrated that electric stimulation at highly selective sites in the brain meant that laboratory animals could be operated on without anesthesia.

Research has uncovered in the last 20 years how morphine acts on the brain, and also found the presence of specific receptors for pain relief on the cells. This led to the exciting discovery of the body's own morphine, the now-famous endorphins. The observation that electrical stimulation of certain areas of the pain pathway could block pain, along with new knowledge of receptor sites, suggests a link. And here it is: The pathways whereby morphine or electrical stimulation produce freedom from pain are precisely the sites of action of the endorphins.

> *Nothing begins, and nothing ends*
> *That is not paid with moan;*
> *For we are born in other's pain*
> *And perish in our own.*
>
> —Francis Thompson

# Painkillers

The more you can learn about pain, the more you can arm yourself against it. Pain goes with the human condition. Some folks seem to have an unfairly large share. In fact, the word comes from the Greek for penalty. Pain is a penalty for all, because it is extremely rare that someone is born completely insensitive to pain. The early derivations of the word are also translated as punishment. In ancient times, pain was perceived as being a punishment for something you did that displeased the gods.

But perhaps compassion is the compensation; when you see someone else suffering, you want to do whatever you can to help. Doctors, as frequent witnesses of anothers' pain, although given many ways to help (some of which don't work well enough), are constantly seeking new and more effective options. For a long time, painkiller drugs have been the answer; however, to be strong enough, they are also dangerous enough to require a prescription and careful monitoring.

Painkillers work by stopping the central nervous system from functioning at its normal level. This is not undesirable when the pain is temporary; but for a long-term chronic condition, it is bad news. We don't mean to say that painkilling medications don't have their place. They do. The opioids such as morphine, codeine, and Demerol can be of crucial, irreplaceable importance, especially with severe traumas, and with post-surgical and terminal patients. But as you know, narcotic analgesics for severe acute pain induce dependence and undesirable side effects; and, over time, as the body builds up tolerance, higher and higher doses may be required to be effective.

The non-narcotic analgesics, especially NSAIDs (non-steroid anti-inflammatory drugs) also come with a price to pay. Although close to 100 million prescriptions are filed for NSAIDs every year (and over-the-counter sales must be even higher), many people don't recognize that they can cause serious problems.

There is evidence of stomach erosions or ulcerations in 40% of those who take NSAIDs for extended periods of time. In fact, it is estimated that over 76,000 people are hospitalized each year for gastrointestinal complications due to NSAIDs. (Each hospitalization costs an average of $10,000.) Last year the Arthritis Advisory Committee unanimously recommended to the FDA that all NSAID labeling be updated to include warnings about the risk of severe gastrointestinal complications.

The occurrence of ulcerations in the small bowel have also been linked to NSAIDs by researchers at the University of Texas. They concluded that small bowel complications of NSAID use requiring surgery may occur more frequently than is currently recognized.

Most people are completely unaware of the dangers of long-term use of common over-the-counter pills for headaches and other kinds of pain. Sometimes the over-the-counter drugs were previously prescription drugs. Sometimes aspirin or other NSAIDs are ingredients in other over-the-counter drugs, so consumers may be getting more than they realize. "It's a public health problem," Dr. Michael Kimmey of University of Washington Medical Center stated at an AMA media briefing in July of 1997. Dr. Kimmey points out that people are so accustomed to these drugs, they take them without really needing to, and without a doctor's advice. A chilling note: People who do come into the hospital with stomach bleeding, warns Dr. Kimmey, have a 10% chance of dying.

Most consumers are also unaware that mixing these common pills, especially acetaminophen (Tylenol), with alcohol represents an even more serious risk: damage to the liver that can be fatal. And what is less well known, they can result in damage to kidneys. A recent article in the *Journal of the American Medical Association* warns against NSAIDs harm to the kidneys. A study was done at the Mayo Graduate School of Medicine in Rochester, Minnesota. The kidney disorders (nephropathy) of at least 10% of patients appeared to be the result of taking over-the-counter or prescription NSAIDs. Even one or two ibuprofen capsules taken two or three days per week can cause kidney problems, according to lead researcher Dr. James McCarthy. And according to Dr. Dominick Gentile, a kidney specialist at Nephrology Specialists Medical Group in Orange, California, and vice president of medical affairs for the American Kidney Fund: "NSAID use, especially in kidney patients, is a real potential problem, and most NSAIDs, even at relatively low doses, can cause other problems such as interstitial disease and tubular necrosis."

Just as we were writing this book, the FDA came out with a proposal to mandate alcohol warnings on all over-the-counter pain relievers. For example, they propose that acetaminophen-containing product labels include this statement: "Alcohol warning: If you drink three or more alcoholic beverages daily, you should ask your doctor whether you should take [product name] or other pain relievers. [Product name] may increase your risk of liver damage." Although at this time we don't know what the result will be, since the public has 90 days to respond, it does illustrate the government's concern.

Cortisone and related drugs given to relieve pain have numerous side effects such as gastric disorders, osteoporosis, increased susceptibility to infections, and even mental disturbances. Even the useful aspirin can cause side effects such as gastric symptoms, tinnitus, allergic reactions, and can interfere with other medications. A Canadian study in 1996 (Tannenbaum) warned that long-term use of NSAIDs should be avoided whenever possible, particularly in high-risk patients such as the elderly. The study warned: "Currently, no NSAID is available that lacks potential for serious toxicity." Some physicians will prescribe antidepressants for chronic pain, and these too have a high incidence of disturbing side effects.

Perhaps some physicians tend to over-prescribe NSAIDs because of the patient's expectations (sometimes called "patient pressure"), or simply because there aren't many alternatives. Another Canadian study found that many physicians prescribed NSAIDs unnecessarily for the elderly. Residents in internal medicine were four times more likely to prescribe an NSAID unnecessarily than were other doctors. This is important, since these are the physicians who are most apt to treat these kinds of patients, and implies that the problem will probably get worse as the residents enter practice. Researchers concluded, and several U.S. medical authorities are in agreement stating that this "raises questions about the appropriateness of NSAID use in the general population."

We have described this problem at some length because the people who might benefit most from magnet therapy are those with chronic pain, such as from osteoarthritis, who may be taking NSAIDs on a long-term basis without being fully aware of the consequences. If they are among the elderly population, they are probably also taking at least two or three other medications for various conditions. The mixing of medications and NSAIDs poses additional risks.

What are their options? Few people will want to go on taking their over-the-counter painkillers if it means they will have to give up having a cocktail or two per day. They can take a painkiller that is less toxic, but also, not as potent. Or they can try a lower dose, but that may bring no pain relief. Magnets, as you will learn, have an excellent track record of safety and have none of these adverse side effects. We hope that learning more about the dark side of painkillers will motivate you to learn more about magnets.

As if pain in and of itself weren't problem enough, it is also expensive—monstrously expensive in terms of medical costs and lost income. Statistics from the American Society of Anesthesiologists: Low back pain disables 5 million Americans and forces them to lose 93 million work days per year. Over 40 million suffer from recurrent headaches, and spend $4 billion annually on pain-relief medications. Arthritis affects 66 million, one-third of whom have to curtail their daily activities because of pain. According to the Department of Health and Human Services, chronic pain costs the national economy more than $79 billion every year and rises to $80–90 billion when you factor in associated legal and health costs. Chronic pain cuts productivity by more than $65 billion. Of course, when you are suffering pain, whether acute or chronic, you don't care about dollar cost or work time lost; you only want relief as fast as possible.

Headaches are responsible for more visits to physicians than any other chronic complaint. Up to four out of five Americans have a least one severe headache a year, and close to half the population have more than one a month. Surprisingly, headache, backache, and other pains seem to occur more frequently in the late teens and early twenties than in other age groups. Some studies link a higher incidence of pain, especially back pain, with increased job stress—a factor far too many Americans have to contend with.

Here is a mnemonic, or memory device for remembering basic pain concepts:

**P:** Pain is a *perception* of personal sensation of hurt.

**A:** Pain is an *awareness* of current or impending tissue damage.

**I:** Pain is an *integration* of impulses to create a pattern of responses.

**N:** Pain is a *negation* of usual behavior, a stimulus response to protect us from harm.

This last is obvious, but important. If we didn't feel pain, such as the burn of a hot stove, we might injure ourselves further. It is indeed a warning signal. In an instant of time too small to be measured, we can pull our hand back from the stove, or our bare foot from a sharp rock. In this sense, we actually need pain for our protection.

Sensing pain to protect us from harm is a particular problem with diabetics, who, due to poor circulation in their lower extremities and neuropathy (nerve disorder), often can't feel when they have cuts or ulcerations on their feet. They may also be unaware of serious infections that develop; in many instances, amputation is required. Oddly enough, diabetic neuropathy can also be characterized by the reverse: severe pain in the feet. There is no successful standard treatment for this. However, in one very recent report, magnets were able to relieve pain in three out of four patients with diabetic neuropathy.

Another problem with pain is that it can be *referred*. Pressure on one nerve can be felt in different locations, say, lower back, thigh, or big toe. An injury to your neck might be felt as a pain in your hand. Referred pain follows specific segments called dermatomes, based on the development of the human embryo. The segments are not all connected, however, thus an injury may not be felt in the original site, but elsewhere. The most common injury sites that refer pain to another part of the body are neck, shoulder, and lower back.

Exercise, vital as it is for maintaining good health, can often produce pain. Continued muscle action over time produces lactic acid, which is a cause of pain. Since pain is primarily an acidic condition, it is likely that the metabolic alkaline/acid balance in the body plays a role in perception of pain, such as the times of the day when pain—perhaps relating to the intake of meals—is worse or lessened. Some believe that pain, in addition to an acidic state, exists in or emits a positive magnetic field, but to date this has neither been proved nor accepted. In point of fact, there is no such thing as an exclusively positive or negative magnetic field, and it is important, both for patients and health professionals, to clear up this confusion, as we will do later in chapter 5.

Pain that is hard to diagnose is too often labeled as having psychological or emotional origin. This kind of pain does indeed exist, and must be treated psychologically. But other kinds of pain may come from a long-standing pattern of tension.

An overload of stress can definitely make these worse. Stress and pain are intricately interrelated. It is apparent that pain is exceedingly stressful and stress can be exceedingly painful. Paradoxically, in some rare cases, such as for a few moments on the battlefield, extreme pain is not felt due to the overwhelming stress. This is probably due to the release of endorphins. During World War II, it was noted that soldiers under the stress of battle conditions, who were severely injured or even had had parts of their bodies blown away, often experienced no pain for several hours. However, this was rarely seen in civilian life when similar damage occurred in a sudden accident.

The "runner's high" is thought to be due to an increase of endorphins which produce a pain-free euphoria like that induced by morphine. Marathoners have even been known to continue running despite having developed bone fractures.

A vivid example of this phenomenon was supplied by the African explorer Dr. Livingston (of Stanley and Livingston fame). In the 1850s he recounted his response to an attack by a lion some 20 years before:

> I heard a shout, and looking half around, I saw the lion just in the act of springing on me. I was upon a little height. He caught my shoulder as he sprang, we both came to the ground below together. Growling horribly, close to my ear, he shook me as a terrier does a rat. The shock produced a stupor similar to that which seems to be felt by a mouse after the first shake of the cat. It caused a sort of dreaminess in which there was no sense of pain or feeling of terror though I was quite conscious of all that was happening. The shake annihilated fear and allowed no sense of horror in looking around at the beast. This peculiar state is probably produced in all animals killed by the carnivore, and if so, is a merciful provision by our benevolent Creator for lessening the pain of death.

# Acupuncture

As a neurologist, Dr. Lawrence specializes in the treatment of pain, and is well versed in pain problems. When he served on the President's National Advisory Council on Aging, he had a chance to observe the problems of long-term pain, especially in the older population. As president of the American Medical Athletic Association, he has learned a great deal about the link between physical activity and pain in people of all ages.

Back in the 1970s Dr. Lawrence started what was probably the first in-patient pain clinic in the United States under the auspices of UCLA. He and his staff treated patients at the clinic with different pain modalities, including acupuncture, which he had recently studied.

Dr. Lawrence even developed some of his own acupuncture techniques, which were later widely used. Other therapies used were TENS (transcutaneous electrical nerve stimulation), psychotherapy, and body therapies such as massage, and the Alexander and Feldenkrais techniques. The clinic was successful in treating many patients. In fact, insurance companies funded the program because they found their people went back to work faster after treatment with the clinic's approaches.

As we noted earlier, the Chinese have for millennia studied the art of healing and relieving pain through acupuncture, and believe it is based on the vital energy (*Qi*) of the body. This vital energy flows through channels called meridians, related to specific organs. Needles are inserted at specific sites where these meridians approach the surface of the body. Some practitioners believe that magnets applied to acupuncture points can mimic the effects of inserting needles, as an ancient Chinese text suggests. The Japanese have tiny *tai ki* magnets that are used for this purpose. Japanese baseball pitcher Hideki Irabu made his debut pitching for the New York Yankees with tiny magnets covering his pitching arm. You can imagine how stressed and sore the muscles of a pitcher's arm must get.

To begin with, acupuncture was scoffed at by the Western scientific community. Although its ability to relieve pain had been recognized for over 4,000 years, it was looked on as no more than quackery. One prominent critic called it "quackupuncture." The turning point came when James Reston, a prominent reporter for the *New York Times,* suffered an attack of acute appendicitis while on assignment in China with President Nixon. The remarkable relief he had from pain during and after surgery, delivered by just three acupuncture needles, led to his famous front-page story. Reston trumpeted: "I have seen the past, and it works."

This led to an explosion of public and scientific interest. Within months, a team of distinguished physicians was dispatched to China to verify acupuncture's benefits for pain and other conditions. The Western doctors were impressed and quickly corroborated many claims, publishing a report in the conservative *Journal of the American Medical Association.* President Nixon's personal physician described how he had seen major surgeries performed with only acupuncture for anesthesia. American newspapers showed photos of Chinese patients cheerfully sipping tea while undergoing open chest surgery, having only one or two acupuncture needles in their arms. There were numerous accounts of people crippled with arthritis who could now walk and run, and totally deaf children whose hearing had been restored.

Dr. Paul Rosch observes that most physicians, himself included, remained cynical. The numerous cases of amazing cures usually came from "barefoot doctors" practicing in remote areas, rather than trained physicians. Their medical records were terrible. Most of the studies showing how acupuncture had relieved asthma or arthritis had no controls, or the diagnosis was questionable. Critics suggested that a large part of acupuncture's popularity was due to the fact that it was a very inexpensive treatment for the millions of Chinese who had little access to other medical care.

It has been said that those who do not learn from the mistakes of history are doomed to repeat them. Let's look at the turnaround that has taken place since Reston's article catapulted acupuncture into the spotlight. Back then, there was no regulation in the field. Many acupuncturists had no formal training, and simply tried to repeat what they had seen others do. The vast majority were non-physician Asian practitioners, accustomed to treating small communities of their compatriots. Because of the huge public demand, they were overwhelmed with patients looking for help and answers. Many physicians were besieged with questions, and became increasingly impressed with what they heard about acupuncture. Some traveled to the Orient to receive formal training. Others went to France or England, where alternative medicine was more widely accepted, and accredited acupuncture training had been set up.

Among these were two good friends of Dr. Rosch, Drs. Norman Shealy and Ronald Lawrence, who were convinced that acupuncture could provide pain relief and wanted to learn how it worked so they could bring it to their patients. Dr. Rosch has always admired their willingness to take months away from very busy practices to live abroad at their own expense in order to learn the procedure properly, and to find some scientific explanation for why it works. Both subsequently made significant contributions to acupuncture as well as to magnetic therapy, based on this educational experience.

# Osteopuncture

Dr. Lawrence began as a general practitioner. In the early 60s and 70s he had many older patients in a nursing home, and every day he saw too much pain taking the joy out of their last precious days of life. Gradually he began to try whatever he could to relieve pain, including biofeedback and behavior modification. He found very few things to offer patients that could really help. When he heard the first news stories about acupuncture's ability to relieve pain coming out of China, he was "turned on." He initially began learning acupuncture back in 1972, studied in Los Angeles with Korean acupuncturists, then in England and Hong Kong.

Dr. Lawrence began to notice that when he used the acupuncture needle on a very thin patient, there was contact with the surface of the bone. Then came the best part: The patients reported less pain when such contact had been made. Pleased and inspired, he went on to develop the technique. Certain areas of bone produced better results. The knee, for example, is painful for many older people, one of their most common problems. The head of the fibula on the outside of the knee turned out to be the right location for reducing knee pain. Sometimes by treating this spot alone, he could reduce pain completely.

More research focused his interest on the bone covering, the periosteum. This smooth bone surface contains many blood vessels and serves as anchor for tendons and muscles. It also has an abundance of nerve fibers.

Osteopuncture is now being taught in Australian medical schools, and in Canada, and is included as part of the acupuncture program at UCLA. It is also taught to Physical Medical residents, and approximately 400 doctors have been trained in the technique over the years since it was developed. It is also taught at several schools throughout the country that train Certified Acupuncturists. As you can imagine, it is most useful in arthritis, with the symptoms of stiffness, aching, and swelling.

Dr. Lawrence feels it would be preferable to try osteo-puncture before considering cortisone, painkillers, or other medications, which often come with unwelcome side effects. The technique is not a cure, but it relieves or removes arthritis pain, and reduces many of the symptoms that handicap so many arthritis patients, such as stiff or inflexible joints.

# The Electro Side:
# TENS, NET, and LEET

Electricity, via TENS (transcutaneous electrical nerve stimulation), brings relief by providing electrical impulses that suppress pain messages from nerve fibers to the brain.

Pain relief via TENS was the achievement of Dr. Norman Shealy along with Dr. Saul Liss, an electrical engineer. Often referred to as "the little black box," it applies electrical energy with specific characteristics to target sites on the body. TENS can be very effective in treating persistent pain. Drs. Shealy and Liss later demonstrated that these effects could even be enhanced by simultaneous brain stimulation with similar weak electrical forces. They also found that this approach could help many patients suffering from depression, jet lag, and other disorders that could be due to low levels of serotonin and other brain chemicals. Not everyone realizes that, although the popular new antidepressant drugs work by increasing brain serotonin, electrical stimulation boosts serotonin more rapidly. Furthermore, the electrical method treatment is safe, cost-effective, and has none of the unpleasant side effects often linked to the drugs.

TENS has long been an accepted treatment for the relief of pain. More powerful, GigaTENS stimulation to selected acupuncture points has recently been shown to remarkably increase levels of the now popular anti-aging hormone DHEA (dehydroepiandrosterone). And unanticipated improvements in patients with pain and other symptoms of diabetic neuropathy not related to increases in DHEA, suggest other important actions that are being intensively investigated by Dr. Shealy. Those who take the "ring of fire" (term for the acupuncture points) treatment report a significant boost to energy and well-being. Some of Dr. Shealy's older male patients reported a marked increase in sexual activity (a welcome side effect).

More recently, Drs. Shealy and Liss have teamed up to develop new instrumentation that seems to produce superior results, and is appropriately called the She-Li TENS device.

Neuroelectric therapy (NET), which evolved from Dr. Margaret Patterson's experiences with electroacupuncture, has produced promising responses in patients addicted to heroin, cocaine, morphine, and amphetamines. Research studies suggest that each of these substance-abuse problems apparently responds best to different parameters of amplitude and frequency. Fine-tuning of these, and correlation of cures with changes in brain neurotransmitters, will likely further improve results.

The addictive pathway from the limbic system to the frontal lobes has recently been delineated, and found to be lined with dopamine receptors. In animal studies, the ability of addictive drugs to provide pleasure and cause cravings disappears when the dopamine-containing neurons are destroyed, or drugs that block their entry into dopamine receptor sites are administered. It is possible to stop an enraged, charging bull dead in his tracks by remote stimulation of an electrode placed in a pleasure center. Could similar, safe, noninvasive strategies be devised to treat drug addiction, stop people from eating or smoking, or help them sleep? Let us hope it will be soon.

Low energy emission therapy (LEET) with the Symtonic device, which creates a weak electromagnetic field in the hypothalamus, already appears to be the most effective and safest treatment for insomnia. This has been confirmed in double-blind polysomnography studies at top university sleep centers in the U.S., in accordance with the strict protocol required for FDA approval for efficacy and safety.

Symtonic LEET has also proven beneficial for the treatment of Valium addiction, anxiety, and other stress-related symptoms, using different emission energies. (The mechanism of action is believed to be mediated by modifications of stress-related neurotransmitter and ion activity.) Sophisticated brain imaging studies show that LEET has a pattern of action almost identical to Valium, but without its side effects or addictive tendencies.

## Auricular Medicine for Pain

The word auricular means of the ear. In France, a major electric and communications company manufactures a tiny magnet that comes in two parts to be used in auricular medicine. The unit is the size of a gelatin capsule. One part consists of a sharply pointed, minuscule magnet that is inserted into the skin of the ear with minimal pressure. The other piece is a small circular magnet which, when rotated over the magnet in the ear, creates a weak electromagnetic field. This stimulates acupuncture points in the ear.

Auricular medicine was discovered by the French neurologist Paul Nogier of Lyons. In the 1950s, Dr. Nogier had a patient with sciatica who had been treated in North Africa by a native healer—a portion of the upper ear was cauterized, which brought instant relief of the sciatica.

Sciatica, a sharp pain running down from the lower back and hip, radiating down the thigh and into the leg, is often caused by a herniated lumbar disk, and is one of the most severe and stubborn pain conditions to treat. Dr. Nogier became fascinated with this patient, since he knew that the outer portion of the earlobe and the external ear canal was supplied by two cranial nerves—the vagus, or tenth cranial nerve, and a branch of the fifth cranial nerve, the trigeminal nerve. After extensive research, Dr. Nogier made an amazing discovery: various areas of the body could be plotted on the ear skin regions. The configuration he obtained almost corresponded to an inverted fetus in relation to our body areas and parts.

Dr. Nogier found that by stimulating certain areas on the ear's "body map," for example the hip area, he could alleviate all or a portion of the patient's pain problem in the hip; or that by stimulating the abdominal area, he could reduce a gastrointestinal complaint. After intensive experimentation, Dr. Nogier plotted over a hundred such points on the ear and earlobe. He began to teach his method widely to physicians in France and Europe, and eventually even taught Chinese doctors. The People's Republic of China honored him with one of their highest scientific awards.

Dr. Nogier and his associates also taught many American physicians the techniques. Dr. Richard Kroening, a former professor in the Department of Anesthesiology at the UCLA School of Medicine, explored auricular medicine, along with his associate Dr. Terrence Oelsen. Many physicians learned the method at UCLA and elsewhere. However, the stringent and necessary scientific double-blind studies needed to gain acceptance of the method by the majority of the medical profession are still largely lacking.

Electrical, acupuncture needle, and magnet stimulation of the points on the ear have been used to treat a large variety of human ills, but mainly for pain. The small French magnets are still widely used in Europe. Despite the loss of Dr. Nogier, who was well into his nineties, his students carry on.

# A Glance at Pain Research Today

All the mechanisms of pain and how they unfold in the human body have not yet been fully charted. The nervous system is slow to yield all its secrets, perhaps because it is incredibly complex, like a dense forest of finer and ever-finer branches.

Some natural substances may be helpful against pain. Substance-P also can be depleted in sensory nerves with capsaicin, the natural pungent compound in cayenne pepper (*Capsicum frutescens*). Capsaicin is a frequent component of some over-the-counter skin preparations to relieve pain. The amino acid DL-phenylalanine also has a good history against chronic pain, especially by inhibiting the enzyme that degrades the body's own natural painkillers, the endorphins. Other promising pain relief substances are sulfur compounds DMSO and MSM.

A new drug made of cone snail venom offers hope as a way to reduce severe pain with very few side effects, and so far, no tolerance or addiction problems. It was presented in 1996 by William Brose, director of the Pain Clinic at Stanford University of Medicine to a meeting of the American Pain Society. Other types of animal venom may also serve this purpose. Several years ago, researchers isolated a painkiller from frog skin that was hundreds of times more potent than morphine. However, it had too many toxic side effects for clinical use. Since its structure was somewhat similar to nicotine, chemists have tried to develop products that would relieve pain without causing other problems. According to a January 1998 report in the prestigious journal *Science,* they have succeeded. A new, nicotine-like compound called ABT-594 appears to match morphine's ability to dull pain, but doesn't have any of the side effects. It also doesn't have the addictive power of nicotine. Safety trials in humans are now being conducted.

One way to stop the pain signal from getting to the brain would be to interrupt its passage in the nerve or nerves responsible for its transmission. This can be done through a surgical procedure called rhizotomy. It may be difficult to accomplish in sites where many nerves are bundled together, like the spinal cord, and nerve roots. Other nerves might be destroyed, resulting in permanent numbness, paralysis, and other problems. A variety of rhizotomy techniques have been used over the years, including trying to pick off only the nerves you are after with a probe that is something like a piano wire.

Radio frequency waves have been used to treat trigeminal neuralgia, or "tic douleureux." This is probably the most severe pain that humans can experience, and has been described as a stabbing or shooting sensation like a white-hot iron. It comes on suddenly, and although it usually lasts for only a few seconds, can recur in paroxysms for minutes, hours, or even days. It can be so violent that patients often become motionless because they are stunned by its intensity. The cause is unknown, and treatment in the past such as trying to inject alcohol was so unsatisfactory that some sufferers even committed suicide. Things have improved today, and one of the safest, most effective treatment approaches is radio frequency rhizotomy. As you can imagine, it is not without possible complications.

During rhizotomy for neck pain, using a tiny radio-frequency generator, surgeons raise the temperature of the tissue surrounding injured, inflamed nerves in the spine and the neck. This procedure literally cooks the tissue and kills the few tiny nerves that sense pain. Dr. Mark Lodico, of the Allegheny General Back Institute in Pittsburgh, says this procedure is most effective on whiplash pain, and that most patients have somewhere between 50% and 100% pain relief. Rhizotomy is also used to treat cerebral palsy and other conditions, such as bladder dysfunction due to nerve damage. In one report where electrical stimulation was used with rhizotomy on nerve-caused bladder dysfunction, 90% of patients had complete relief (Van Kerrebroeck, University Hospital Nijmegen, The Netherlands).

In the next chapter, we will examine how magnets can be used to alleviate pain. But let us note here a striking similarity between where magnet therapy for pain stands today and where acupuncture was thirty years ago. Magnetic therapy suffers from the same lack of early standardization, scientific credibility, and regulation. Yet look at what has happened with acupuncture. To obtain a license, most states demand evidence of certification requiring three years of formal education that must include 1,350 hours in clinical and classroom training. The majority of the 15 million patients who have turned to acupuncture are now treated by physicians.

In November 1997, acupuncture was recognized as a valid, worthwhile therapy by the National Institutes of Health not for pain, but for the nausea associated with chemotherapy. A twelve-member panel gave an official endorsement, and one of the doctors pronounced on national television: "It's time to take this seriously."

A recent study, funded by the R. W. Johnson Foundation and reported by *USA Today,* noted that among 4,124 deaths, families reported that 40% of patients died while in severe pain for almost all of their final days. Most people, as they head through middle age toward the last part of life, say that they fear pain even more than they fear death itself. This attitude must change as the older segment of the population grows larger. Physicians need to deal with disabling pain with strong measures, and we should not allow fear of addiction to increase the suffering of those who have been declared terminal. Studies indicate that when patients are allowed to control the frequency and amount of pain medication through intravenous dispensers, the medication is not abused. In fact, according to the *Encyclopedia Brittanica,* some reports show that less medication is used than would have been prescribed.

But the fact remains that chronic pain does not have to be an inevitable part of growing old. With new techniques and old techniques such as acupuncture, osteopuncture, and magnet therapy, most pain can be alleviated and brought under control. Pain is also highly variable as perceived by different individuals, some having a higher pain "threshold" are able to withstand it better. Part of this may be due to cultural factors, childhood experiences, gender, and so on. But it is important to remember that the mind does play a key role, both during and after, in how pain is perceived.

Dr. Lawrence observes:

> The amazing aspect of pain is that it is forgotten. The wonder of the human mind is that once it is over, pain falls through our memory and is forgotten like water running through a sieve. But our joyous moments, our pleasures, are caught and held.

And Dr. Rosch likes this quote from *Paradise Lost:*

> *The mind is its own place and in itself*
> *Can make a Heaven of Hell, a Hell of Heaven.*
>
> —John Milton

# Magnets and Pain

*We are the mirror, as well as the face in it.*
*We are tasting the taste, this minute,*
*of Eternity. We are pain, and what cures pain, both.*
*We are the sweet cold water,*
*And the jar that pours.*

—Rumi

**P**ain is the foremost medical motive for the use of magnetic fields. So, for a first-time user, whether patient or physician, it's important to understand some of the mechanisms involved, even though science still hasn't pinned down or confirmed all of them.

Dr. Lawrence feels that the optimal use of permanent magnets is for chronic pain. (Pain is considered chronic when it has been fairly persistent for at least thirty days.) Dr. Rosch is equally impressed with the ability of magnets to relieve pain in patients with acute injuries, or transient arthritic complaints, and has reported on the success of magnets in reducing bruising and inflammation following plastic surgery.

Dr. Lawrence estimates that today in the United States more than 200,000 people are using magnets; that number could be more like 2,000,000. Some claims estimate that magnets can help as many as 98–99% of all patients if properly used. In the personal experience of Dr. Lawrence, over 80% of his patients have shown at least some (and sometimes maximal) response to the use of permanent magnets. He considers 80% not only satisfactory but amazing.

Let's pause for some very important points. Magnets should only be used when a diagnosis has been made to identify the cause of pain. Remember that pain is a warning signal that must be respected. Do not try to treat your own chronic painful condition without having consulted a qualified health practitioner. Magnets should not be used when the cause of pain is uncertain. Furthermore, in our view, magnets should not be used to replace medications that may be more appropriate or even necessary. Rather, think of magnets as often highly useful adjuncts that enable people to reduce drug treatment, thus minimize unwelcome side effects.

In chapter 5 we will tell you about the different types of magnets and where they should be placed for best results. Today's powerful but small magnets can provide significant relief for the aches and sprains that are so common for everyone—more specifically for sore muscles, muscle spasms, and minor injuries of athletes, the painful arthritic joints of the elderly, and the wrists and necks of computer operators.

## How a Skeptic Became a Believer

His reputation as a pain specialist brought Dr. Lawrence together with magnets at an unlikely place—the world of the race-track. Dr. Lawrence would label himself "conservative," having treated thousands of patients over forty-five years as a physician; he's also seen all kinds of medical trends and fads come and go. When he first heard of magnetic therapy, his reaction was "some kind of quackery." Then he became personally involved when he received a referral from the Los Angeles County Medical Association, an organization for which he had been an advisor in many instances regarding alternative health practices. Now they referred him to a magnet company that had a history of manufacturing permanent magnets, mostly for use by veterinarians for treatment of horses. The company had an excellent track record using magnets on pain and arthritis—not only for horses, but also for riders and trainers. This skeptical doctor was invited to do an infomercial. They wanted him to talk about pain, however, not about magnets.

He did so, and then his curiosity took over. Could magnets really be a new and valuable therapy? The president of the company gave him papers to read by British, German, and French authors and scientists on magnets. As time went on, this skeptic became a believer—albeit a very cautious believer by virtue of medical training, and the fact that so many so-called remedies that come up the healing pipeline turn out to be spurious and not backed by any hard scientific evidence. What turned the tide for Dr. Lawrence were the results he experienced after treating his own patients with magnets. He became so excited that he urged other physicians—including top-notch orthopedic surgeons, some from major universities, many in the California area—to try the magnet approach. Lo and behold, every one of them found that patients benefited to some degree by the use of permanent magnets. In 1991, to learn even more about how magnets worked and how best to use them, Dr. Lawrence founded the North American Academy of Magnetic Therapy, a forum where interested doctors and scientists could present their findings. The Academy has become a center of information exchange with doctors and researchers from all over the U.S. and around the world.

## The Electromagnetic Aspect

There are differences between what permanent magnets and electromagnetic therapy devices have been shown to do, and more importantly, what they have been proven to do in regard to various conditions. Drugs and devices cannot cite any medical claims unless they have passed stringent FDA standards demonstrating safety and efficacy.

This can be a double-edged sword. The regulations are designed to protect the public from drugs and devices that have not been thoroughly tested for long-term or unsuspected side effects. (Remember the thalidomide tragedy years ago that caused so many tragic birth defects?) On the other hand, the FDA system may deprive the public from having easy access to useful therapies that are readily available in other countries, having passed similar rigid testing there. Further, testing to satisfy FDA protocols can be a lengthy and very expensive process.

At present, proponents of permanent magnets in the U.S. are not allowed to make any claims, including pain relief, even though they have proven to be effective in double-blind studies for at least two types of pain and are completely safe. It is likely that FDA approval will be sought for certain applications in the near future, as additional double-blind studies are reported.

Electromagnetic field therapy has shown to be effective in numerous disorders, but is approved only for the treatment of bone fractures that have failed to heal normally. This was largely due to the efforts of Drs. Robert Becker and Andrew Bassett, who were pioneers in studying the effects of electromagnetic forces on regeneration and healing processes. They did extensive animal studies to prove their theories before attempting clinical trials to show that magnets were safe and effective.

Several electromagnetic devices are approved for healing fractures, and have been successful for hundreds of thousands of patients, including some with fractures that had failed to heal for fifteen years or more. A side note of interest: Once the FDA has approved a drug or device for one condition, physicians are free to use it for any other, because safety is not a concern. Many pharmaceuticals are prescribed for "off label" indications that later become approved. For example, when Inderal first became available, it was only approved for angina. However, it was probably prescribed more for hypertension; since it was so effective for that condition, it quickly became another accepted indication. So you see, electromagnetic devices are now often used to treat depression and pain, promote soft tissue and fracture healing, and alleviate a host of other complaints, even though such claims cannot be made.

Another fact to keep in mind is that FDA approval simply means that certain claims can be made by the manufacturer on the label or for promotional purposes. Prior to 1976, no approval was required for any medical device, and there were all sorts of weird electrical machines on the market making claims for pain relief, baldness, sexual rejuvenation, and so on. Anybody could make and use these devices.

There was a crackdown after 1976. Only devices like diathermy, which had been used for years by physicians and hospitals, could continue without passing rigorous and expensive testing procedures. The same occurs when a new specialty is established, and certification is sought without proof of adequate training and experience. Physicians who are well established as cardiologists are usually "grandfathered in" without taking tests, as long as their practice record shows they are qualified. This "grandfathering" can provide a loophole for some devices. If, for example, examiners can be convinced that a device is essentially the same or very similar to a diathermy machine in current use, it may not have to satisfy the usual requirements for new devices. And once it has received clearance, it can be used for other purposes, as long as no claims are made. Devices that provide weak electrical stimulation to the brain have been used to treat pain, insomnia, and depression; one manufacturer recently won a lengthy court battle with the FDA, which had cited him for promotional claims they felt were unjustified.

# European Research

Dr. Rosch's involvement in this arena came from his interest in electromagnetic field therapy. An internationally recognized authority on stress, he had been approached 15 years ago by Swiss scientists to evaluate the Symtonic device they had invented for treatment of stress-related complaints. They showed him extensive animal studies and clinical trials they had performed in Europe demonstrating that the device was safe and significantly improved anxiety and insomnia due to stress. Dr. Rosch was impressed with the data and their thoroughness. He encouraged them to do further research to explore the mechanism of action—how it worked.

Dr. Rosch visited the Biotonus Clinic in Montreux, Switzerland, supervised by Claude Rossel, M.D., Ph.D. The facility was devoted to offering patients the best of two worlds: the most reliable methods that alternative medicine had to offer, plus sophisticated space-age medical technologies and approaches. Previously, Dr. Rossel had directed research for a major Swiss pharmaceutical concern and was a trained investigator. He had become increasingly interested in non-drug approaches. In conjunction with nearby medical centers, he thoroughly investigated placental therapy, which was popular in France to promote healing; anti-aging procaine therapy in Romania; and fetal cell injections, which originated with the work of Dr. Paul Niehans in Switzerland. All these therapies had strong anecdotal support, but little scientific validation.

Drs. Rosch and Rossel became good friends. Dr. Rosch helped to guide the Symtonic research and acted as Medical Consultant to the Clinic. With Dr. Rossel's encouragement, he organized the First International Montreux Congress on Stress in 1988. It attracted leading authorities in various areas of stress from all over the world, and many sessions were devoted to electrotherapeutic approaches. These included presentations by Dr. Bjorn Nordenstrom on his theory of the body's electrical circulatory system, and a remarkable treatment for metastatic lung cancer based on this; Drs. Norman Shealy and Saul Liss on cranioelectrical stimulation for treating depression and jet lag; an update on the Symtonic research by Drs. Rossel and Rosch, and other cutting-edge advances.

Of particular interest were the sessions devoted to what might be called "electromedicine," often chaired by Dr. Ross Adey, probably the world's leading authority on the effect of electromagnetic energies on the brain. Distinguished authorities from Europe, Russia, Eastern Europe, and Japan have also presented exciting research studies over the past ten years. These have included not only electromagnetic devices, but scientific studies of mystics and healers. Japanese investigators showed sophisticated imaging studies in patients undergoing acupuncture and electroacupuncture. At the 1997 Congress, more than two days were devoted to this unusual research, as well as to advances in magnet therapy. A presentation showed for the first time that application of a permanent magnet could significantly increase levels of beta-endorphins, the body's own painkillers. This increase took place in an hour or so, which could explain why some magnetic bracelets can relieve pain in areas far from the wrist.

# Mechanisms of Pain Relief from Magnets

So, exactly how does it happen? How can a magnetic field reduce pain? Dr. Lawrence believes that perhaps the main actions are relaxation and circulation. Magnetic fields appear to greatly increase blood flow in the tiny capillaries. For example, via testing by plethysmography, a way of measuring blood flow through the fingers, Dr. Lawrence found a rate of 300% increase in five minutes—a dramatic change. The speeded circulation is thought to be due to the relaxation of capillary walls and important changes in the capillary beds, as well as further relaxation of muscle and connective tissue.

Capillaries are key to understanding how magnets relieve pain via increased blood flow. The capillaries, far narrower than arteries or veins, are the regulators of blood flow. They are turned off until there is a need for carrying oxygen in and carbon dioxide and other waste products out. Then they are activated. Blood flow in tissue is governed by how many capillaries are flowing, just as water use in your home depends on how many faucets are opened. When their walls are relaxed, they allow the blood to flow more freely.

The relaxation factor has led to the invention of magnetic massaging devices. These produce a gentle relaxation of smooth muscles, and Dr. Lawrence observes even some skeletal musculature has been noted to relax with the use of permanent magnets.

Capillary action helps pain in another way: by speeding up fluid exchange in injured tissue, thereby flushing away the pain and inflammation chemistry at the site. These include unwanted byproducts such as lactic acid, which are major causes of pain and inflammation. It is as though the life processes in the affected area were suddenly made more efficient once unwanted fluids were flushed from the system. In most cases, this stepping up of the metabolism not only stops pain but also stimulates the body to heal faster since the movement of oxygen and other nutrients to the cells will increase as the capillary blood flow continues.

## Fields in Motion

Dr. Rosch believes the mechanism of action may occur at a more basic level. He states that magnetic fields can produce no biologic effects unless there is motion in the field. Electromagnetic fields are always in motion, but the only things we can see that are moving in a static magnetic field are blood and lymph. However, there is a constant invisible motion of ions as they pass in and out of cells, and good reason to believe that this is where "the action" is—in both static and electromagnetic fields as well as enzyme systems, especially those that affect the production of ATP (adenosine triphosphate). As will be explained later, ATP is the source of energy for all cellular activities.

An ion is an atom or group of atoms with a positive or negative charge. Sodium, calcium, potassium, and magnesium are positive; chloride and phosphate are negative. Like magnets, opposite ions are attracted to each other, which is why we have, for example, sodium chloride, or salt. Positive ions like potassium and calcium compete with sodium to get hooked up to something negative. Electrical activity results because of the motion of these charged particles, which in turn are affected by magnetic fields.

Permanent magnetic fields, as well as those from electro-magnetic devices, are unique in that they pass freely through all body structures, just as if they weren't there. Heat, sound, electricity, and x-rays are blocked by bone, are slowed down by skin resistance, or absorbed when they encounter soft tissue and muscle. Magnetic fields sail right through everything, and can easily reach deep-lying structures such as nerves that transmit pain signals. This could include the sciatic nerve, solar plexus, and all of the brain.

Dr. Lawrence believes there is also an alkalinizing effect, since pain is primarily an acidic condition. The acid/alkaline balance of your body is of key importance. The fluids around the cells are meant to be slightly alkaline. Too much acid (naturally produced by your cells as they function) must either be neutralized or eliminated, or toxic conditions are created for the cell.

## Magnetic Versatility to Be Explored

The ability of magnetic fields to provide so many diverse clinical benefits suggests their modus operandi is at a very basic level of cellular function. This appears to be confirmed by research studies demonstrating that they alter the dynamics of calcium, potassium, sodium, and other ions transport across cell membranes. In turn, these can have profound effects on essential enzyme systems that influence ATP formation.

When you think of ATP, think energy. These phosphate bonds ultimately provide the fuel for every single cellular function in the body. Since both electromagnetic and permanent magnet fields can influence ATP activities, this could explain certain common attributes, and would seem a rich area to explore. For example, electromagnetic therapy for cancer and cardiomyopathy is clearly enhanced by manipulations of sodium and potassium ionic flux designed to affect ATP.

Here's a provocative thought: Could certain nutritional supplements or interventions also improve magnet therapy? Is there a way to demonstrate this in the laboratory? Why not nutritional support? After all, the ancient Chinese believed that herbals enhanced the power of lodestone therapy.

Similarly, if motion is a prerequisite, could the effects of permanent magnets be enhanced further if they were constantly moved over the site of application?

Earlier views on the mechanism of electromagnetic fields and circulation continue to be debated. Some still claim that magnets attract the iron in the hemoglobin molecule, and this increases the flow of blood. There is absolutely no evidence to support this, or reason to suspect that it is true. The iron in hemoglobin is in a bound form, and has no magnetic charge or capability of being influenced by a magnetic field.

Others point to the magnetite present in human brain tissue. This has been contested, but a couple of recent studies back up the magnetite theory. Some feel this theory may have some merit. A 1996 study out of the University of Western Australia at Perth confirmed the existence of magnetite in some brain cells by examining tissue from patients during brain surgery. But at present, Dr. Rosch has no convincing evidence that magnetite is involved in any way in magnetic healing.

However, theories aren't important, only facts are; and the indisputable fact is that magnets do work. Let's look at a few of the common pain applications.

# Arthritis Pain

---

Arthritis is one of the very earliest diseases. We have the proof, via x-rays of mummies, that arthritis existed among the population of ancient Egypt. Alas, it will hit us all sooner or later. Everyone over 60 will show arthritis on an x-ray, even if the symptoms are mild to nonexistent. For most sufferers, however, the various forms of arthritis are not mild but manifest in troublesome symptoms such as aching, swelling, stiffness, and actual pain. Of the 66 million people diagnosed with arthritis, according to *USA Today,* one-third of them have to curtail their daily activities because of pain.

Arthritis is essentially a bone and joint disease. About 80% comes in the form of osteoarthritis, a degenerative condition based on the wear and tear of just living. Rheumatoid and rarer forms of arthritis, such as psoriatic, make up the rest. And let us not forget gout—represented by that laughable picture of a fat monarch of centuries past with his throbbing foot up on a stool. But it's no laughing matter for the sufferer. About 100 different disorders can give rise to arthritis, including gout caused by urate crystals deposited in the joints. "Pseudogout" (no less painful for the "pseudo" term ) is characterized by inflammation from calcium phosphate crystals. Arthritis can also be triggered by systemic disorders such as lupus and inflammatory bowel disease, and can result from rheumatic fever, tuberculosis, Reiter's syndrome, gonorrhea, and Lyme disease.

In all of Dr. Lawrence's practice, the greatest use of magnets is for the treatment of pain from degenerative (or osteo) arthritis. The wear and tear can affect any joint along the spine, in the neck, the lower back, knees, elbows, wrists, or fingers. He has had remarkable success in using magnets for the pain caused by these conditions. He has even had good results in cases of TMJ (temporomandibular joint disorder—a real jawbreaker of a label!), which causes sharp jaw and facial pain. Spondylitis with its stiff, aching neck also responds well to magnet therapy.

Whatever the cause or symptoms, the key to arthritis is pain control. There is no such thing as a real arthritis cure because the degenerative changes are irreversible, and the calcium deposits will remain in the joints. Magnet therapy, reinforced by lifestyle changes of improved nutrition and regular exercise, can go a long way to making arthritis bearable.

## *Case History: John D.*

John D., a 40-year-old, hard-working, high-powered executive, came to Dr. Lawrence with a two-year history of low back pain. He had played football in high school and been injured several times. An MRI examination showed degenerative disc disease with no frank herniation at the L-45 and L5 S-1 levels. The pain involved went down the back of his legs to the knee areas. He was having great difficulty adjusting to this in his busy life.

He was given a brace containing ceramic magnets. He wore the brace whenever his pain bothered him, about two or three hours a day. He was advised not to wear it constantly or it might cause a weakening of the back muscles. In addition he used a magnetic pad with neodymium magnets on his chair at the office. As he does with all patients who begin to use magnets, Dr. Lawrence gave John some additional suggestions. This ancillary help is always important. For example, he recommended massage and encouraged John to use a little footstool that could be adjusted to help lower back pain. John has not had to use the brace as much lately; but puts it on when he gets an acute episode. And when he travels on airlines, he always wears his magnetic "corset."

### Case History: Les W.

Les W. was 60 years old. He had pain from the degenerative type of arthritis in the fingers of both hands. A part-time machinist who loved to sculpt and paint in his free time, Les was a man who needed full use of his hands. He was given wrist magnets made of neodymium. In addition, for his fingers he was given neodymium dot magnets, held in place by cotton gloves to be worn at home and at night. This controlled his discomfort up to about an 80% level. Les, otherwise in good health, liked to ride bicycles but found gripping the bars uncomfortable. Wearing the gloves with the neodymium dots, he was able to grip much better. Four years later, he still wears the gloves to get relief, with periodic breaks to accommodate the body's adaptation mechanism. He still gets about 80% effectiveness, sometimes more, depending on the weather, he says. In cold weather, it's more difficult.

### Case History: Fiona Y.

Fiona Y., a lovely 84-year-old woman, otherwise in reasonably good health, had bilateral osteoarthritis in both knees. There was pain, particularly in the medial portion. The swelling was marked—her knees were about four times the size of normal. She was trying to be active, but because she couldn't use her knees properly, wasn't being active enough and had put on extra weight. This is a common problem. People who are inactive tend to add weight and this actually makes their condition much worse.

Ceramic magnets were used in a special type of knee gauntlet of neoprene to hold them in position. Amazingly, overnight her knees reduced in size by 200%. In the following days, as she began to move about and the tissues could pump out the fluid, the swelling reduced even more. Within a week her knees were almost back to normal size. They couldn't become completely normal because of the degenerative arthritis in the knee joints, but she was extremely happy to have 90% relief of pain. She found that when she experienced a lot of activity, she might notice the effects the next day. However, she did wear the magnets at night, and still does so.

## Headache Pain

One of the most widespread complaints is the headache. Although there are many varieties, and with multiple causes, the chief trigger of headache pain is constriction of blood vessels, hence decreased circulation. When blood flow is restricted, it's somewhat akin to a garden hose with a kink in it. This produces the pain sensation. The constricted area will not be receiving oxygen, so that hypoxia (oxygen starvation) occurs. Many people today who work at computers and sit for long hours in the same position will develop tension-type headaches. The neck muscles are stressed without adequate rest. These types of headaches will respond well to permanent magnets, with their action of increasing circulation to the target site.

The migraine headache is a different situation, believed to involve constriction and then dilation of blood vessels around the brain, promoting release of substances (neuropeptides) that act to further increase swelling and inflammation. The causes of migraines seem to include a genetic tendency, fluctuating hormone levels, and stress.

Approximately 80% of people with headaches are female. Wearing magnets (the earlier ceramic or the later neodymium type) around the temporal areas and at the back of the head have brought fair results in relieving tension headaches.

### *Case History: Katharine T.*

Katharine T., a 34-year-old office worker, suffered headaches classified as the muscle contraction or tension type. They occurred on a daily basis. When she wore the magnets as directed in the evening hours, it would alleviate about 50–60% of her discomfort. Dr. Lawrence also gave her a Relax Band with a neodymium magnet over the wrist, which helped reduce her tension. She described her job as "high-stress," but felt after the headache relief and the Relax Band that she was able to handle it.

# Post-Surgical Pain and Healing

The results achieved by Dr. Daniel Man confirm that applying a permanent magnet pad following liposuction surgery markedly reduces bruising and inflammation, and promotes healing. There is a notable reduction in post-operative pain, so that patients require less pain medication. He has had similar results in reconstructive and other plastic surgery at his Surgery and Laser Center in Boca Raton, Florida. There has been a marked increase in demand for such procedures, especially by aspiring models, who find being able to return to work more rapidly and have fewer post-operative problems important. Dr. Man feels he has shortened the recuperative time by 50% or more in most patients, and believes this is because the magnets improve blood flow to the affected area providing more oxygen and nutrients and removing toxic waste products. The photographs on page 177 show the effect of the magnetic pad following abdominal liposuction.

Dr. Marko Markov, visiting Professor at the Mount Sinai Medical Center in New York, believes that magnetic and electromagnetic fields have profound effects on a number of body processes, including musculoskeletal injuries and wounds caused by surgery or trauma. He estimates a success rate of approximately 80% with virtually no reported complications.

# Pain of Injuries

Permanent magnets have long been used in the world of horses, whose tendency toward leg injuries (sprains and fractures) is well known. Millions of dollars are spent on magnets for horses, but then horse racing is a lucrative business. What's good for the horse is also good for the trainer, owner, or rider. One of the most famous horse trainers of all time, Charles Whittingham, whose statue welcomes visitors to Santa Anita Race Track in California, swears by permanent magnets for his lower back. He has worn them for years. We will return to equine therapy later in chapter 9.

## Magnets and Pain

Injury to muscles during sports activities is a constant. Whether it's golf, tennis, football, or baseball, many athletes are now firm believers in magnets and wear them taped to the area of sprain or strain. They find magnets especially useful to calm muscle spasm. Jim Colbert, senior PGA Tour golfer, is one enthusiastic fan of permanent magnets. He smacks out a line drive or sinks a delicate putt with magnets strapped to his lower back. Don't tell him magnets are placebos. He thought his career was over a few years ago, when he couldn't play more than three or four holes without excruciating back pain, which also affected his swing. Another golf professional, by coincidence an old friend and patient of Dr. Rosch, suggested Colbert try magnets based on his own personal experience. Colbert scoffed at the idea but agreed to give it a try. He went out the next day with magnets strapped on his back, played eighteen holes with little distress, and almost won the tournament. The rest is history. He was the leading money winner on the 1995 Senior PGA Tour ($1.4 million), beating the likes of Jack Nicklaus and Arnold Palmer.

In 1996 he was tops again ($1.6 million, a new record), and was voted Player of the Year. People couldn't believe that he was a "cripple" in 1994. Colbert attributes his success entirely to magnets, and has stated publicly numerous times that he could not play golf without them. Senior tour player Bob Murphy and LPGA star Donna Andrews have stories that are equally dramatic, and their public praise is just as lavish. Over 70% of the senior tournament golfers are believed to use magnets, although not all admit it, often because their agents want them to get paid hefty sums for promotional advertising using their name, and some have such arrangements. The amazing thing about Colbert, Murphy, and Andrews is that they receive absolutely no reimbursement for their enthusiastic endorsements because the particular manufacturer refuses to do so. However, they are so grateful for being able to resume their careers pain-free, that they consider this more than adequate reimbursement for their comments to the press, and even display the company's logo on their bags for the fans and television audience to see.

Denver Broncos linebacker Bill Romanowski uses a magnetic mattress pad to relieve pains acquired from the constant battle crunch of the football field. Henry Ellard and Leslie Shepherd, receivers for the Washington Redskins, rely on magnets for pulled muscles. Chris Jones of the San Diego Padres uses magnets on a regular basis. Baseball players in Japan have been taping small magnets onto their sprains and aches for two or three decades.

Ryan Vermillion, head trainer of the Miami Dolphins, swears by the use of magnets to keep the players off the training table, and on the field. For over two years the team has been using magnets for aches, pains, and to promote healing. After injuries, players are able to return to the field faster due to the dramatic reduction in pain and swelling, thanks to the application of magnets. Star quarterback Dan Marino's broken ankle was supposed to keep him sidelined for two months, but Vermillion gave him magnets to use and he was back in weeks. Vermillion believes the magnets increase the flow of oxygenated blood to the injured area. The Miami Dolphins are so sold on magnets that they recently purchased a magnetic pad for the players to sit on during games when they are not on the field, which also prominently displays the manufacturer's logo. Not only Vermillion, but also all the players, swear by magnets as well. Many team members have purchased magnets for personal or family use.

## *Case History: Richard K.*

Richard Kearney, a retired lawyer in his sixties, developed a sudden severe pain in his left shoulder and could hardly lift his arm. An MRI test confirmed that he had a tear in his rotator cuff muscle. He was told that he would most likely need to have surgery if he didn't improve after a month of physical therapy and medication. Kearney is an avid golfer, has a home with several acres adjacent to a golf course in Great Falls, Virginia, and maintains the property himself with a good-sized John Deere tractor that does not have power steering. He became more depressed as he watched his golfing buddies out on the course from his porch, and quickly found that it was impossible for him to even maneuver the tractor without pain. Dr. Rosch suggested magnet therapy.

Treating the shoulder is often difficult because it is a large area, and motion may cause the magnet to change position. Dr. Rosch was able to obtain a new undershirt designed specifically for this purpose. Made of a lightweight fabric that dries three times faster than cotton, it is a variant of that used for magnet therapy in horses, who sweat a great deal when they run. Both shoulders have a pocket sewn in which allows you to slip in a 4" × 6" thin and flexible pad containing fifteen powerful magnets.

Kearney was skeptical, but his pain was so severe, even with medication, that he agreed to give it a trial for a day or two. His pain had progressively lessened by the time he went for his usual therapy session five days after putting the magnet on. The therapist couldn't believe his increased range of motion, especially since he was now taking little pain medication. Kearney was told to continue using the magnet and to report back in a week. The improvement continued and the tractor now posed no problem. When he returned for his next visit, he had no symptoms. The therapist had never seen anything like it, and called the doctors in to verify the improvement themselves since they were unlikely to believe his written report.

Following their careful examination, Kearney was told that not only would surgery be unnecessary, but he could stop coming for therapy and resume normal activities cautiously. The following day he was back playing eighteen holes of golf, and soon found that he could even carry his bag if necessary. Dr. Rosch later received a letter saying: "Before I started wearing the magnet, almost any movement caused pain, and after, no pain. Maybe it's more mind over matter than magnet, but I don't care. The result is immense relief: no surgery and freedom from pain. In fact, even my other shoulder (right) which has troubled me from time to time, feels much better. I don't know why. I just know it does." When Dr. Rosch spoke with him eight months later, he had experienced no recurrences, was playing at least eighteen holes a day whenever he could, and carrying a bag was no problem.

### Case History: Jennifer T.

Jennifer T. was an attractive single woman in her mid-thirties who worked in a small office, not only typing but packing. It was in grabbing a falling box that she injured her right hand. Stretching of the radial nerve caused a neuritis that brought pain to the back of the thumb, running up the forearm on the lateral side. The pain meant that she was unable to do her work or sleep well at night. She described herself as "at the end of my rope."

Dr. Lawrence placed neodymium magnets along the course of that nerve; within a few days she had 80% relief from pain. Over a period of weeks, she used the magnets less as her body began to heal itself. She soon was relieved to find herself back to normal and with no residual effects.

## *Case History: Nancy J.*

Nancy J. was very active at age forty-five, a dedicated runner. She stumbled while out running one day and injured the inside of her left thigh. There was a severe sprain of the adductor muscle. After spending weeks at the usual therapy of ice, massage, and the over-the-counter NSAIDS (non-steroid anti-inflammatories), she was getting nowhere.

When she came to Dr. Lawrence, two months after the original injury, she was fed up with the constant pain. She was eager to try anything, and magnets sounded good. Her primary benefit came from a checkerboard pattern flexible magnet, gauss strength 450, applied within an ace bandage. Only fifteen minutes after the magnetic field was applied, she noticed a decrease in the pain; by the next day, the pain was virtually gone. She continued to wear the magnet for two weeks, then gradually returned to her running in stages, starting with bicycling. Four years have passed with no return of the problem.

These are only a few of the potential applications of magnetic fields for pain. If your health problem has not been covered here, look to chapter 6 for further applications of magnets to various types of conditions and disorders, and the late-breaking and future developments discussed in chapters 8 and 10.

# CHAPTER 5

# Magnetic Devices and Their Placement

- Doctor to Doctor
- Magnetic Devices
- How Long to Wear Magnets
- Strength
- Patterns
- Magnets and Acupuncture Against Stress
- The Window Phenomenon
- Polarity
- Making Better Magnets
- Magnets in Motion

W hat type of magnets should you use in what situation? Where do you place your magnets for best results? Understandably, doctors and patients may both be confused. Dr. Lawrence feels that placements are crucial in the effective use of permanent magnets, and that placements take precedence over the type of magnet being used or the polarity. Proper placement of magnets can produce effects, whereas wrong placement may not. Table 5 compares the differences of magnetic field distribution between single poles of magnets and a bipolar magnet.

The following section is intended as a guide for physicians or appropriate health professionals. Others might want to skip forward to learn about the different types of magnets available.

# Doctor to Doctor

There are three major placements for magnets in therapy: local, at the area of referred pain, and the acupuncture points. The local method involves placing magnets right over the pain site. A typical example of referred pain is a problem in the hip, in which the pain may be referred to the knee. The theory is that if you treat the local area, such as the hip, you don't get as good results as you would from treating the referred area, for example the knee. Dr. Lawrence believes it is best to treat both areas.

Acupuncture points have been found to be effective (see chapter 1, figure 1.1). Often, when magnets haven't been successful at pain relief over the local or referred areas, then using them at the proper acupuncture points will frequently bring results. Sometimes the referred area is the same as an acupuncture point. The practitioner should keep trying all possible combinations until pain relief is achieved.

### *Headaches*

With headaches, surrounding the scalp with magnets can help. Magnetic fields go right through bone to the brain: The skull

**Table 5   Measurements of Magnetic Field Distribution at Various Distances**

| Distance | Single Pole | Single Pole | Bipolar |
|----------|-------------|-------------|---------|
| Surface | –1109 | –847 | –273 |
| 0.25 | –727 | –525 | –183 |
| 0.5 | –494 | –386 | –104 |
| 0.75 | –354 | –227 | –61 |
| 1 | –257 | –162 | –39 |

*All distances are in centimeters and the magnetic field is expressed in gauss. Readings from two single pole magnets of different strengths and bipolar magnet in the last column.*

does not stop transmission of magnetic waves into the brain. The treatment of headaches with magnets though seemingly effective, still needs further investigation.

## *Joints*

When dealing with a joint, such as the wrist, knee, hip, or ankle, try placements on all sides of the joint. Toe problems are best handled by magnetic inserts in the shoe, but the inserts must be powerful enough. They are more effective if worn directly against the skin, although they can penetrate adequately through the material of a sock. For the toe, it would be best, if possible, to surround it with magnets. It's effective to treat the ankle from two sides, but four is even better. Knee placements should also be at the sides, but again, including the front and back is even more effective. Some companies make wraps that cover all four sides, which work best for treating the knee. If you have a choice of covering only two, then do the medial and lateral (middle and outside) rather than front and back.

## *Hips*

The hip is a difficult joint. You want to surround it as much as possible. A good local placement is over the bone that protrudes at the side of the hip, the greater trochanter. One placement over that can be effective. Hip arthritis can be uncooperative, however, and does not respond as well to permanent magnets as does the knee, for example, or the elbow.

## *Spine*

Most of the magnets for the spine are made to be worn over the spine or lateral to the spine, hitting the acupuncture as well as the local points. Dr. Lawrence has found that when it is possible to get a magnet over the abdomen and over the back, the overall effectiveness is increased.

## *Shoulder*

For the shoulder, placement on the front and back is most effective.

## *Neck*

Because it is hard to put magnets in front of the neck, using them lateral to the spine and over the spine if possible seems to work. If you have only one choice, use magnets lateral to the spine, which happens to coincide with acupuncture points along the Bladder Meridian that parallels the spine. The point

Bladder 20 is located at the soft area where the skull meets the neck, laterally, where you feel that soft depression just beneath the skull bone. This is an effective area, not only for neck pain but for headache, and worth placements on both sides.

### Elbow

If you can surround the elbow in four places, fine; if not, at least make placements over the bones at the lateral and medial portions. These are called the epicondyles.

### Wrist

Use front and back placements for the wrist. By surrounding the pain site, penetration occurs on all sides; that has worked best in our experience.

# Magnetic Devices

---

The permanent therapeutic magnet is often encased in ceramic or embedded in an elastic patch or flexible strip. Permanent magnets are also used in wrist supports, back supports, seat pads, and as strips to be worn inside shoes. Magnets can be made of metal, ceramics, or neodymium (a rare earth metal), and each type is claimed to be superior for certain situations. The neodymium gives a deeper penetration.

A popular form is a rubberized permanent magnet that can be cut into different sizes and shapes to apply to different parts of the body. "Plastiforms" with magnetic strips are particularly handy because they can be molded around a joint or part, and easily cut with scissors. Besides ceramic and "plastilloy" types, there are the rare-earth magnets, chiefly using neodymium. Some of these types originally came from the world of industry, where they were used for car motors, refrigerators, electric motors, and so on. These, of course, were not designed for therapeutic use; that is why you will occasionally find strange gauss strengths in certain magnets.

Among the new devices, wraps have become very sophisticated. A wrap is important because it brings the magnet right against the skin, and also makes it comfortable to wear as needed and as frequently as can be managed—sometimes all day long. There are different kinds of wraps—some made of cotton or new nylon material; some breathable, some rubberized for knee and elbow.

*We cannot emphasize enough the importance of magnets being close to the skin.* Because there is a logarithmic falloff of strength relative to the air space between skin and magnet, the objective is to keep the magnet adhering to the skin. Many can be taped on. We suggest using the paper tape made by 3M that is used medically. Even adhesive tapes are satisfactory or an ace bandage can be added to hold it on better.

Dr. Rosch cited in the last chapter a case of a painful torn rotator cuff, the muscle in the shoulder. The question for the sufferer was how to apply a magnet and keep it there while moving the arm. Dr. Rosch is enthusiastic about the results received with the special T-shirt for shoulder pain (see figure 5.1). It has pockets for magnet insertion over the upper spine, which can be another difficult area for proper placement. He feels that if motion indeed increases the effectiveness of a magnet, then this might be better than strapping one in place with adhesive, since slight changes in position occur with body movements.

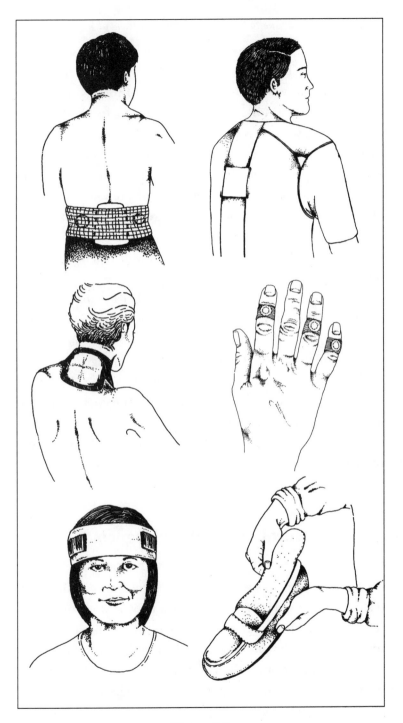

**Figure 5.1**

Pads and mattresses are also available. These can be expensive, but have multiple benefits such as pain relief and restful sleep, as we will describe in some of the research studies. How do they work? Magnets embedded in blankets, pillows, and mattresses may be several inches from the body's surface, and their relationship to any specific acupuncture site keeps changing. Their effectiveness suggests that benefits do not depend on precise placement or field strength, which falls off with the square of the distance from the patient. These sleep pads, many with quilted covers, are placed on top of the mattress. Mattresses are also made with magnets embedded in them.

The reason mattresses may work is because of the much greater number of magnets used as well as their stronger gauss strengths, thus, both factors may overcome the lack of skin contact and the lack of local or acupuncture siting.

Dr. Dean Bonlie, a dentist from Calgary, Alberta, in Canada, tried sleeping on a mattress with magnets to relieve lower back pain and found it successful. He now designs magnetic mattresses and claims that they improve sleep. He has presented no hard scientific data on this, but he states it will be forthcoming soon.

## How Long to Wear Magnets

Dr. Lawrence believes that you can wear magnets all the time. It's perfectly safe. However, we suggest they be worn until pain relief occurs. Then they can be taken off, and if pain should return, they can be put back on. It is advisable to remove them when you shower or take a bath. Of course, any device should be used according to the manufacturer's suggestion.

After a period of three weeks, Dr. Lawrence feels the magnets should be discontinued for three days. A physiological phenomenon called adaptation, which is based upon homeostasis, represents the body's attempt to come back to balance. This can be achieved in a period of about three weeks—sometimes more quickly, sometimes more slowly. So when the body has adjusted to the magnetic forces in the fields, the effectiveness may be worn down. This happens with drugs, for example. Adaptation is Nature's safety factor to help us achieve stability in case we're exposed to toxins. Surprisingly, we can frequently adapt to toxins, which is shown by the fact that children who live in a smoggy environment have an actual adaptation as the body starts to protect itself.

This is why we suggest taking a break at the end of three weeks, for several days at least, then resuming magnet use. Many times people discovered that if magnets were losing their effectiveness, after a break from using them, the magnets regained effectiveness. On the other hand, Dr. Rosch knows of patients who have worn magnets continually for longer periods of time without losing their effect. Also, in one recently reported double-blind study on diabetic neuropathy, patients wore magnets continually night and day for four months (since results often are not seen until after six weeks or more in many patients). Among Dr. Lawrence's patients are some who have worn magnets for four or five years, especially those with arthritic conditions. However, he has them take periodic breaks.

Dr. Lawrence, who has followed up on patients over time, obtained results of at least 80% effectiveness with magnets. This is a remarkable figure. As another means of assessing the situation, his office watches the magnet return rate. That is, patients are told they will get their money back if they are dissatisfied and return the magnets. The return statistics help to show what response people have to the magnets. To date, the overall return rate in Dr. Lawrence's office, which involves several different magnet companies, has been 3%.

Dr. Rosch has also noted the considerable confusion and controversy concerning the site of application. Some practitioners believe that magnets activate acupuncture points and meridians, and that they can be just as effective as acupuncture for certain complaints. In Japan, tiny *tai ki* magnets have been designed to directly stimulate acupuncture sites with pinpoint precision.

Magnetic bracelets are used to prevent or relieve pain in various parts of the body. Since no clear correlation exists between these locations and meridians in or near the wrist, there is little reason to assume that their effectiveness is due to an acupuncture-like effect. The same applies to necklaces, rings, and other magnetic jewelry. If such items do indeed produce analgesia at sites where there are no detectable field effects, it may be that magnets provide information as well as energy, and that such subtle signals are not as distance-dependent as thought. There is good evidence that the benefits are not simply placebo effects. However, much less is known about how these benefits are achieved, or how this energy can be measured.

## Strength

The strength of permanent magnets is described in units of gauss, or tesla, with one tesla equaling 10,000 gauss. (A magnetic field of one gauss is about twice the average magnetic field at the earth's surface.)

Every magnetic device has a manufacturer's gauss rating, but its *actual* power below the body's surface is usually much less. For example, a 4,000-gauss magnet transmits only about 1,200 gauss to the patient. Indeed the effective gauss strength is less again, as the strength falls off quickly at greater depths inside the body. The actual strength of a magnet also depends on its size and composition, making many gauss ratings meaningless and misleading.

Therapeutic magnets use from 200 gauss up to perhaps 1,500 gauss, which is only a fraction of what an MRI machine emits. Compare this to a less than 10-gauss magnet on the refrigerator that holds the shopping list or the kid's drawing.

## Patterns

Some pads employ a pattern based on some patented geometric arrangement of contiguous opposite polarity zones such as checkerboard patterns, circles, parallel lines, or packed triangular forms. The manufacturers tend to claim that they work because of an engineering principle known as the Hall effect, and that such patterned magnets have a greater ability to produce biological benefits not obtained by other types of magnets. However, we do not believe this is the correct explanation, and no conclusive evidence exists to back up these statements. The adequate performance of these pads is most likely based on the fact that the gauss levels are multiplied by the geometric configuration.

With certain of these patterned magnetic devices, because of the flexible nature and frequent bending, re-examination will reveal entirely different and jumbled patterns months or years later. The problem with this is that patients may not get as good results, and therefore will become discouraged about magnets and not benefit from their use. It is not clear whether this is entirely due to repeated physical bending, or to the natural tendency for magnetic fields not to stay in artificially created domains. It is a minority of scientists at present who feel that patterned magnets may not work as effectively as other types of magnets.

A Swiss scientist named Arno Latske designed an alternating polarity magnet in 1981, and found that it demonstrated a beneficial effect when placed over an area of pain. This design was further improved by Horst Raermann of Germany, who used alternating concentric rings. Most recently, Vincent Ardizone, an American, developed a new magnetic pole design that uses a triangular pattern. Each cluster of triangles has four sides with different polarities adjacent to poles of opposite polarity. He feels this configuration mathematically increases the probability that a blood vessel will cross alternate poles. We present this information for the knowledgeable reader, but we must emphasize that no good scientific studies exist to prove statements that these magnets are superior as therapeutic tools. The companies that manufacture these magnets state that definitive studies are planned.

## Magnets and Acupuncture Against Stress

Anxiety and stress are far too prevalent today. Most people prefer not to use tranquilizing drugs to control the problem—their lives are too busy, and they must remain mentally alert. Yet anxiety leading to stress can impact the body in many negative ways. The chief culprit is the adrenal hormone cortisol, which at excess levels has been blamed for promoting degenerative diseases and premature aging.

Dr. Lawrence realized that stress was behind most visits to his office, and for years he looked for a weapon that would be safe, inexpensive, and effective. He hoped to find a way that would not hurt the body, and eventually looked to magnets. The result: a tiny but powerful neodymium magnet, 1,500 gauss, encased in ceramic, sewn into a flexible, elasticized band. The band is worn on the inside of the wrist over the acupuncture point P6 (also called *Nei-Kuan*), which is associated with stress reduction. This point has been used by Chinese acupuncturists for thousands of years to induce a sense of tranquillity.

When the wearer snaps the Relax Band against the skin of the wrist, impulses go up the sensory nerve tracts to the brain and into the thalamic area. From here the impulses are relayed to the limbic system at the front of the brain, the primary area in which emotional responses evolve. With this relay message, the chain of anxious thoughts is broken. The wearer can note the stress-related sensations in the body decrease and frequently disappear. Anxious thoughts, which tend to become chains of thoughts, are stopped in their tracks. This mechanism, described by the famous Russian scientist Ivan Pavlov, is called a conditioned reflex, and can change cerebral patterns.

There are two separate mechanisms at work here: The magnetic field created by the small magnet in the flexible wrist band exerts its force on the P6 point and acts to chronically reduce stress due to an *acupuncture* phenomenon.

# The Window Phenomenon

How can a tiny magnet, small as a dot, bring about real benefits? To scientists and laypeople alike, it seems impossible that the small electromagnetic force provided by a fixed magnet can produce a great effect via its energy fields. The window phenomenon helps to explain this effect—that more is not necessarily better. In the case of a tiny dot magnet, there may be a specific window where the magnetic field exerts optimal effects, and energies above or below are not as good or don't work at all. The work of Dr. Ross Adey demonstrated that physiologic responses were obtained only within certain parameters having to do with such things as amplitude, frequency modulation, and carrier signal characteristics for electromagnetic fields.

Dr. Marko Markov's research suggests that an optimal window for permanent magnet effects is about 400–500 gauss *in the tissue, not the magnet.*

Some of the permanent magnets used to relieve pain may be up to 5,000 gauss. That may be necessary if they are in a mattress and at some distance from the body. However, when applied directly, they may achieve no better effect than magnets of only a few hundred gauss.

How many gauss penetrate the human body? As we said earlier, unless the magnet is held really close to the skin, you lose magnetic power in a logarithmic fashion. You don't have to go many centimeters away before you have virtually no field, no matter what the strength.

Basically, the essence of the window phenomenon is that smaller forces can sometimes achieve better results because they fit through the window better.

# Polarity

Dr. Rosch and Dr. Lawrence emphasize that a strictly unipolar or separate positive or negative field is impossible. All magnets have both a north and south pole by definition. These can be readily identified by allowing the magnet to swing freely in a horizontal plane, and determining which end points north, or by seeing which end of the compass is attracted to it. "Positive" and "negative" are also misleading and inaccurate terms that originated with the British Admiralty's efforts to improve the compass. They had created a freely floating magnetic needle mounted over a card containing markings to indicate gradations in direction based on the orientation of the needle when it pointed to the geographical North Pole. The end of the needle that pointed north was called the north or positive pole of the magnet. Actually, it should have been called the "north-seeking" pole, which would have meant that it was actually negative rather than positive. By the time this error was recognized, the terminology had become so ingrained that it was too late to correct it. Similarly, the term "unipolar" is still in wide use and not likely to disappear. It simply refers to the application of either pole to the body, rather than both poles.

Various claims are also made by different manufacturers with respect to the superiority of their product design, or the benefits of applying either pole or both poles to the body. However, there is absolutely no clinical evidence that these magnetic fields produce any biologic effects that are superior, safer, or even different.

## Making Better Magnets

Can permanent magnets be improved, not only to be stronger but to have better or different biologic effects? It's an intriguing question. Various attempts have been made to make magnets more powerful—with success. The permanent magnets currently used to relieve pain are 100 times stronger than those available earlier in this century. In addition to iron, they customarily contain the rare earth metal neodymium and the mineral boron, both readily available and therefore cost-effective for commercial use. Including other rare-earth elements, as Professor Wolfgang Ludwig of Germany did for his therapeutic electromagnetic device, might make them more efficacious. Professor Ludwig has had thirty years of experience in this area. His latest device has over sixty different elements in its iron core, so that he can obtain different resonance frequencies by varying the energy input. In that way, he can target the field to specific organs or sites that have different *resonance* characteristics. We'll discuss this important subject at greater length in chapter 10, where we will explain how magnets can make a frog fly.

It is well known that when certain dissimilar metals are joined together, or touch the body, a minute electric current is generated. As you saw in chapter 2, Galvani first discovered this by accident. Volta proved this by placing some tin on the tip of his tongue, and then touching it with the handle of a silver spoon that touched the back of his tongue to complete the circuit. And Faraday explained why this could be predicted based on atomic weights and electron transfer. (This electric charge can occur from metal dental fillings in your mouth, since several types of metal are often used.) Combinations such as gold/silver, copper/zinc, nickel/copper, or gold/aluminum have this property, which has been termed the "polarity agent effect." Special magnets made in Japan have an aluminum/gold or a nickel/copper insert in their center to provide a small electric current as well as a magnetic field. Others have an aluminum disc protruding from the surface of the magnet to be applied over the acupuncture point to take advantage of *acupressure* as well. Patients are encouraged to gently press or rub them frequently to increase stimulation.

Magnets containing certain metals are said to produce different effects. According to the manufacturer, gold and copper "tonify," silver and zinc "sedate," and titanium and stainless steel "balance." It is not clear in Western usage specifically what these terms mean, or what evidence supports such claims. However, we will see in chapter 10 that different elements have nothing to do with their gauss ratings or physical strength might change the biologic effects of magnets.

# Magnets in Motion

Since motion is an important determinant of biologic activity, it would seem likely that constantly moving any magnet over the treatment site should improve results. Various types of small receptacles containing magnets that can move freely back and forth inside have been designed and marketed. For example, massaging wands and pods provide enhanced pain relief, according to an impressive number of anecdotal reports. The vibrating, moving magnet appears to throw a deeper field. The "pods" look like a peapod, with magnets encased in a plastic sheath. Most other "moving" devices are more expensive and cumbersome to use. Dr. Lawrence has had good results with these pods. When they are placed on the chest in a sheath, they can often relieve the bronchial spasms of asthma sufferers. One of the major uses, for lower back pain, works by decreasing muscle spasm.

Dr. Lawrence also says that if you roll magnets over a site, or hold a vibrator over it, obviously you get a double effect.

You get the massage relaxation plus the magnet effect. The research in this area is sparse, but we do know that a moving magnetic field appears to work more effectively. These are especially helpful with muscle spasms, because the action helps to relax and lengthen the muscle.

It is the gauss strength being delivered in the tissue of the affected area that is crucial. This depends not only on the gauss rating of the magnet, but on its size and shape, and whether both poles or only one is being applied. (You might say that "your gauss is as good as mine"!) Is the composition of the magnet also important? We don't know that yet, but there is reason to suspect that it might.

However, what is just as important as gauss level in the tissue is the *volume* of the field—that is, not only the area covered, but also to what *depth*. Dr. Rosch believes that bipolar products are not as effective because they do not penetrate as deeply, and has studies to prove it. Application of one pole of a neodymium magnet seems greatly superior with respect to penetration, and area can be determined by the size and shape of the magnet to fit a specific application. He compares their relative effect to the difference between a shotgun and a rifle.

Innovative design and application are offering biomagnetic therapy in new forms, the useful mixed in with the weird. Here's a tiny sampling: "Face-lift" masks to beautify the skin (that actually may help with sinus problems), necklaces supposed to increase longevity, even erection enhancers. Special cups manufactured in China claim to reduce dental tartar (and this may be so). Magnetized water and cups used in Japan for almost a decade carry the claim of helping mediate hypertension and diabetes. With all the options and the blizzard of claims, sorting the useful from the weird may seem like a daunting task. We hope that your common sense and this book will guide you well.

Finally, an important point for both physician and patient: When choosing magnets, do not be discouraged if the first attempt proves unsuccessful. Think of the use of medications— when drug A fails to control a particular problem, then it makes sense to move on to drug B.

Suppose that when penicillin was discovered they tried up to 200,000 units without success then discarded it. They didn't know that over a million units might be necessary. Or what if a doctor tried penicillin for a fever, and since it didn't work, assumed the patient didn't have an infection. But the bug might be resistant to penicillin, and another antibiotic would have worked.

So, if a magnet manufactured by company A doesn't work, it doesn't necessarily follow that a magnet from company B would also fail. Sometimes a magnetic product will turn out to be unsatisfactory, perhaps by faulty design or insufficient gauss strength. Some claim the checkerboard or concentric-ring bipolar application produces superior results compared to application of one pole only of a neodymium or ceramic magnet, but this remains to be proven. That is why we suggest that you always ask for scientific studies to support any claims, as well as, a 30-day, money back guarantee. Legitimate companies should always be willing to do this.

It's important not to give up if you don't get instant relief. Some patients do get excellent results within hours or even minutes, but it often takes days or longer for many. When people with back pain hear senior golfer Jim Colbert's story, they give up when nothing happens in two days as it did for him. Five days or a week is more likely to bring results for many patients. Sometimes the relief is gradual, and can only be appreciated by comparing how one feels today to how one felt one or two days (rather than one or two hours) before. And remember the penicillin story. The current magnet treatment might not be getting a strong enough field to the right place, or another product might do the trick.

In summary, when it comes to the placement or the type of magnet, our advice is this: *Keep trying.*

# CHAPTER 6

# Magnets and General Health

- Wound Healing
- Carpal Tunnel Syndrome
- Stress
- Stress-Buster
- Depression
- Fibromyalgia
- Asthma and Allergies
- Arthritis
- Insomnia and Other Sleep Disorders
- Fatigue
- Back and Spinal Disk Problems
- Diabetic Neuropathy
- Magnets and Health Around the World
- Homeostasis and Magnetic Deficiency
- Let Nature Be Your Healer

*Healing is a matter of time,*
*but it is also sometimes a matter of opportunity.*

—Hippocrates, *Precepts I*

Thus here can be great rewards in learning how magnets work and why they can relieve pain and promote health. In this chapter we will cover the versatility of magnets and the many different conditions and disorders for which they have shown benefits.

First of all, what about overall health? When you come right down to it, good health depends on good communication. Our ability to stay alive requires constant maintenance of body temperature, heart rate, blood pressure, and the blood levels of sugar, salt, potassium, magnesium, calcium, as well as proper acid/alkaline balance and so much more. Whenever any of these factors are disrupted or threatened by some stressful challenge, there are automatic natural reactions to correct the situation. These responses have been exquisitely honed over the lengthy course of human evolution.

The status of all functions essential to preserve health is continually being monitored so that integrated endocrine, immune, and nervous systems can return things to normal. This can only be accomplished by some continuous capability that enables us to send instantaneous messages back and forth all over the body on a millisecond to millisecond basis. Electromagnetic pathways?

We have no control over this perpetual process, which is automatic and seems to involve communication pathways about which we know little. But it may be possible for us to take advantage of these communication channels in certain situations. We still can't explain in scientific terms how a spontaneous remission seems to be associated with a strong faith, or why certain healers can cure cancer and other seemingly fatal disorders, or even how the placebo effect actually works.

But such phenomena seem to be consistent with an emerging model of some sort of electrical circulatory system not unlike the ancient concepts of *Qi* and *prana*. Magnetic fields seem to represent a very similar force, and pass freely through bone and all other body structures as if they were air. No other form of energy does this.

As to claims that magnets can cure a disease or disorder, Dr. Lawrence is cautious about the word "cure." He feels this term is unsuitable, that "cure" means there is absolutely no trace left of the original disease being treated. He doesn't think "cures" happen even with drugs or other forms of medical treatment, including surgery, but believes that a physician can alleviate a condition to the point where the patient is no longer troubled with it. Over the passage of many years, say a decade, without reoccurrence of the symptoms or problems, then the word "cure" would be appropriate.

Having planted that caution flag, let's proceed to look at the many applications permanent magnets can have in human health.

# Wound Healing

Dr. Lawrence recalls that as far back as 1960, an experiment by W. J. Erdman, reported in the *American Journal of Orthopedics* (Vol. 2, 1960), showed the magnet-induced increase in blood circulation also increased the number of white blood cells as well as macrophage activity. This creates a bactericidal effect on inflammation and infection, for example, in a wound site. The macrophage (literally "big eater") activity helps to remove waste products and cellular debris more efficiently, and the increase in fibroblast activity and collagen formation results in more rapid tissue growth and, thus, restoration to normal.

Since then, several other studies have reported similar findings, although most of the permanent magnet research dealing with this issue has been done in Eastern Europe, Russia, and Japan. Some of the best examples are Vardanian's research on blood flow, Mileva's on changes in lymphocytes, and Nakhilnitskaia's extensive investigations on the long-term effects of a constant magnetic field on numerous aspects of function as well as composition. However, these are in Russian journals that are not readily accessible; and if they were, would require translation because even abstracts in English are not available. Fortunately, Drs. Pawluk and Jerabek have summarized important Eastern European contributions. Information on how to obtain this is provided in chapter 8, which discusses Dr. Pawluk's presentation at the 1998 meeting of the North American Academy of Magnetic Therapy.

Dr. Rosch was particularly impressed by two cases reported by Dr. Richard Rogachefsky, orthopedic surgeon of Jackson Memorial Hospital in Miami, Florida. The first was a 70-year-old white male who was shot at close range through his thumb. In surgery, all dead soft tissue and bone was cleaned out. An x-ray after surgery showed the complete destruction of the first metacarpal and trapezium (bones) with the thumb completely unstable. A week later an external fixator was placed across the thumb and wrist to stabilize the thumb, and bone was grafted to the crest where the missing bones would normally have been. Five days after surgery, a permanent magnet was placed over the graft, and left there. Within five weeks the graft had consolidated and the wound completely healed. The external fixator was removed, and the thumb was completely stable. Usually a healing of this kind would have taken two to three months. The rapid healing was attributed to the magnetic field stimulation of bone and bone graft.

A second, equally impressive case involved a 54-year-old man who had been in an automobile accident that injured his right wrist. Because of severe and persistent pain, he underwent surgery to remove arthritic portions of one bone, and to fuse four others together to provide stability. This necessitated taking some bone from his hip for a graft. The bones were then held in place by two screws and two wires, and a cast was used to immobilize the wrist. Five days later, a neodymium magnet was placed over the operative site and remained there throughout the course of treatment. This type of four-corner bone fusion usually takes two to three months to heal so that the screws and wires can be removed. With this patient, an x-ray less than six weeks after the operation showed that fusion had already taken place. The screws and wires were removed without incident.

Dr. Rogachefsky's firm impression is that, in both patients, the remarkably accelerated healing of bone grafts and soft tissue injuries came from the stimulation provided by the neodymium magnets.

The experience of Dr. Daniel Man, a plastic surgeon in Boca Raton, Florida, who found that this type of magnet also significantly reduced inflammation and bruising following liposuction procedures, will be shown in chapter 8.

## Carpal Tunnel Syndrome

Carpal Tunnel Syndrome affects thousands of persons who spend many hours each day working at a computer. The constant, repetitious movements cause stress and inflammation to the nerves, resulting in pain and a numbness in the thumb and first two fingers. There is often difficulty in grasping objects, and the pain in the hand can disturb sleep at night.

Many physicians now call it Repetitive Stress Injury, but it is hardly new. In his *Treatise on Diseases of Workers* published in 1700, the Italian physician Ramazzini referred to the "harvest of diseases" that affect workers because of "certain violent and irregular motions and unnatural postures of the body." More than a century ago, *Gray's Anatomy* described a deformity of the hand known as "washerwoman's sprain." Today we also have "pricer's palsy" in store clerks, "Nintendonitis" in video game addicts, and "pickle pusher's thumb" in workers at food-processing plants, where the last pickle must be placed in the jar manually.

Using the word "stress" to describe this condition, as in Repetitive Stress Injury, may be more serendipitous and accurate than is generally appreciated. Certainly the pain and discomfort adds to job stress. A three-year study done at the request of the Communications Workers of America union and U.S. West, a regional telephone company, evaluated the incidence of this syndrome in some 500 video display terminal operators. Information was also gathered as to the quality of workplace life, revealing that carpal tunnel syndrome was most apt to occur in workers with higher stress levels, especially if they felt their work activities were being monitored by superiors. This syndrome has become the highest workplace cost, and often accounts for more than a third of the $60 billion in workers' compensation payments paid annually. It occurs more frequently in those who have higher stress levels because of problems at work or at home, and, in this study, symptoms were present in one out of four workers.

Dr. Lawrence examined twenty-two patients who had mild or moderate carpal tunnel syndrome (to return to the more popular name), as determined by electrical studies—called nerve conduction velocity studies. He and his staff measured the motor distal latency and sensory distal latency times. In this procedure, electrical current is put into the median nerve. The median nerve goes through a fibrous tunnel, enters the hand, supplying sensation and motor ability to certain small muscles in the hand mostly at the lateral portion, and also supplies sensation to the fingers, particularly the thumb and first two fingers.

When repetitive stress leads to carpal tunnel syndrome, it is due to increased pressure on the median nerve through that tunnel. Measuring the electrical changes that occur, you can find a slowing in the electrical transmission. If you put pressure on any nerve, a slowing takes place.

Dr. Lawrence used magnets over the wrist area, after first measuring the transmission times. When the person had worn the magnet for a minimum of six weeks (up to twelve weeks), Dr. Lawrence re-measured and found improvement in twenty out of the twenty-two patients. He never published this study, but it convinced him that something important was taking place.

In view of his experience and clinical observations of many practitioners who followed up on this, he learned that wearing a magnet around the wrist area will help prevent the onset of carpal tunnel syndrome in those who are susceptible (those with repeated use of the wrist). In other words, the magnet is an important aid for *prevention*.

However, Dr. Lawrence found that magnets are not that helpful when a person has advanced or severe carpal tunnel syndrome. In some cases, surgery may be the only answer. To repeat, wearing a magnet at the wrist area is worthwhile as a preventive, since it is both inexpensive and safe.

Four years ago Dr. Lawrence did another study that involved measuring the blood flow through plethysmography. Blood volume was measured and charted in the forefinger. When a magnet was placed on the wrist, he found a 300% increase in blood volume in the forefinger after five minutes. He used strong magnets, at approximately 450 gauss on the wrist area. Again, this is an unpublished study, but has been duplicated by others.

## *Case History: Mark*

Mark, a 45-year-old newspaper reporter who typed furiously on his computer, all day every day, developed pain in the hand and wrist area. The symptoms were fairly recent, about two months old. Dr. Lawrence gave him wrist magnets—now usually made of neodymium, but in this instance they were ceramic. Mark wore them while typing and also at night. Within one week he had 50% relief. Within two weeks he had 90% relief. He also learned some ergonomics that helped him use his wrists with proper support. Through this combination, he was able to achieve virtually total relief. Four years later, he still uses magnets and is still pain-free.

Dr. Rosch supplies these case histories from Dr. James Owens of Lexington, Kentucky.

A 48-year-old housewife with a history of chronic but intermittent carpal tunnel syndrome had been doing well until her symptoms flared after intensive gardening activities. She had severe pain in the forearm and numbness in the thumb, index, and second fingers. She had previously been able to obtain relief with a splint worn while sleeping, to prevent nerve compression. However, at this time, even though she wore the splint continually, her complaints persisted and the pain didn't respond to over-the-counter painkillers. Another week of wearing the splint and taking a stronger analgesic produced no improvement.

Then a neodymium magnet was inserted beneath the splint over the affected area. Within thirty minutes, her pain subsided significantly, and steady improvement followed. The numbness in her fingers disappeared after several days. Three weeks later she was still comfortable. She reported that one night she forgot to wear the magnet and the pain rapidly returned, but went away as soon as she put the magnet back in place.

A 38-year-old female secretary had a history of carpal tunnel syndrome from prolonged typing. Cortisone had been injected locally to relieve her numbness and discomfort, yet she continued to need medication for relief of severe pain, despite regular wearing a splint. Surgery was advised, but she refused to consider it.

A neodymium magnet was inserted beneath her splint at the right location, and over the next few weeks she had a progressive and remarkable reduction in her pain and all other symptoms. She is very pleased with her improvement, continues to wear the magnet, and no longer needs pain medication of any type.

These patients were seen by Dr. Owens in July of 1997. Dr. Rosch checked with him six months later for permission to include these reports, and to obtain follow-up information. Dr. Owens said that in both instances, the patients were now pain-free. Neither had required magnets for several months, except for rare instances when symptoms started to return and the magnets gave prompt and effective pain relief. Dr. Owens also mentioned several other patients who had shown remarkable improvement with magnets, including a man with severe and puzzling pain in the leg and knee, as well as some swelling. The only consistent relief this man could get was with a neodymium magnet. However, if the magnet were removed, and he engaged in normal activities, the pain returned. What particularly impressed Dr. Rosch is that Dr. Owens is no ordinary physician. He has three Board Certifications including one in Pain Medicine and one in Emergency Medicine so that his observations carry special weight.

## Stress

Stress comes in many forms, from physical challenge to mental anxiety. A stress situation causes the secretion of adrenal hormones, which prepare us to meet emergencies; but when these emergencies go into constant overload, the same hormones can cause serious damage over time. Stress is the major trigger of illness, both mental and physical. Dr. Rosch has spent many years studying the impact that stress has on our lives and our health. He has been involved in stress research since 1951, when he began his close association with Dr. Hans Selye, the legendary father of the stress concept. Dr. Rosch has served as president of the American Institute of Stress for twenty years, and has written extensively on almost every aspect of the relationship between health and stress. He is recognized internationally as one of the leading authorities on this subject, even to the point where a German science writer recently referred to him as "the Pope of stress."

Both Drs. Rosch and Lawrence very strongly believe human lives could be healthier and extended by years with simple reduction of stress. Job stress, for example, has reached epidemic proportions and is growing. The vast majority of Americans perceive they are under much more stress now than they were five or ten years ago. In a 1992 survey, one in three reported feeling under "great stress" on a daily basis. In a 1996 poll, almost 75% said they experienced "great stress" on a daily basis.

The relationship between job stress and heart disease is apparently so well known that in New York, Los Angeles, and many other cities, any police officer who suffers a heart attack on or off the job is assumed to have a work-related injury, even if the attack occurs while the person is on a fishing vacation.

## Stress-Buster

As we described in the last chapter, Dr. Lawrence designed a magnetized band to be worn over an acupuncture point that would fight stress. The sensory message from the magnet impacting the wrist point can also stop pain for some people, by stimulating the nerve pathway to the thalamus in the brain. The thalamus, as we said before, is a sort of headquarters for pain, receiving and sending messages. The message also goes to the limbic system, where emotions such as anxiety, fear, and anger are centered.

Dr. Lawrence tested the Relax Band on 200 patients. They were given self-assessment tests, the Minnesota Multiphasic Personality Index Anxiety Scale, and the Beck Anxiety Questionnaire. Results were gratifying: 85% showed clear-cut measurable anxiety reduction, 10% showed some improvement, and only 5% showed no improvement. As of this writing, thousands of people have used the band, and reports from patients and medical colleagues continue to support the anti-stress benefits of using the band.

For years Dr. Lawrence has been a psychiatrist as well as a neurologist. He has found that reducing stress can be the beginning of the ending for a depressive state. Use of the band has given many patients a way out into a more positive state, feeling good about life and about themselves. By the way, the Relax Band is a godsend for people who practice meditation as a way to relax and cope with stress. According to anecdotal reports, stimulating the "tranquillity" point with the magnetic field also appears to help with nausea, whether due to pregnancy or travel motion.

# Depression

Dr. Rosch strongly agrees with Dr. Lawrence about the relationship between stress and depression, and has written a great deal about this. Like the chicken and the egg, it's sometimes difficult to tell which came first, since one can cause the other. Anything you can do to break up this vicious cycle will improve both. Far too many people are walking around with undiagnosed depression. Close to one out of ten of all primary care outpatients suffer from major depression, but only one-third to one-half were correctly diagnosed by their doctors, according to a 1993 report from the Agency for Health Care Policy and Research. The incidence may be even higher, but because of some stigma attached to mental illness, depressed patients are often coded or listed as having a different diagnosis.

There is growing evidence that the majority of depressed patients may suffer from a biochemical disorder over which they have little control. However, three out of four Americans believe that mental illness is purely an emotional disorder, and almost half think that the problem is entirely the patient's fault, according to a study from the National Institute of Mental Health. More than one out of three actually feel that depression is "sinful," and possibly a punishment for past transgressions, a throwback to a notion that was prevalent in earlier times.

Depression is common to all races, ages, and ethnic groups. The average age of onset is in the late twenties, with episodes generally lasting six months or longer if not treated. In addition to the tremendous costs to the health care system, 50% of patients with severe clinical depression eventually take their own lives, and at least 60% of all suicides can be attributed to depression.

In 1990, close to $44 billion was spent in direct and indirect costs for the treatment of depression. This is even more than was spent for the treatment of coronary heart disease, and the figure is expected to surge sharply over the next five years. We can comprehend this trend even more by noting the sales of the highly popular antidepressants: $610 million in 1989, $900 million in 1992, and an anticipated $2.2 billion by 1999!

Many of the drugs used to treat depression are also effective for several other stress-related disorders. The newer drugs act by increasing serotonin levels in the brain. However, the side effects for Prozac can include nervousness, anxiety, agitation, insomnia, nightmares, sweating, anorexia, weight loss, loss of sex drive, and, occasionally, a manic state.

Electromagnetic brain stimulation of varying types has been used with success in the treatment of depression. The mechanism of action is not clear, although studies show that one type of transcranial stimulation boosts serotonin levels, much like Prozac and the newer antidepressant drugs. A very recent new form known as rTMS, or repetitive transcranial magnetic stimulation, may work in a different fashion than those which involve placing electrodes on either side of the head. This new technique is aimed at a specific area of the brain with a hand-held device, and has been found to be extremely effective in depressed patients who were resistant to drug treatment. You'll learn more about this in Dr. Rosch's presentation at the 1998 meeting of the North American Academy of Magnetic Therapy in chapter 8. Of course, electric shock therapy was the standard treatment for severe depression for decades, and is still used in patients who don't respond to anything else. However, this magnetic therapy treatment as well as cranioelectrical stimulation are quite different from the old method. They are safe and cause no discomfort. Whether permanent magnetic fields can also relieve depression is not clear. There are numerous anecdotal reports, but no scientific studies we know of, and some of these unsupported claims seem extravagant. We feel strongly that depressed individuals should always consult a physician.

We mentioned earlier the use of magnets by Tibetan monks, and there are numerous anecdotal reports about the therapeutic benefits of magnets and lodestones to relieve depression. Unfortunately, no scientific research had been conducted to assess the validity of such claims until recently.

Dr. Rosch offers this intriguing follow-up: In an attempt to verify the claims of the Tibetan monks, a carefully designed double-blind study was carried out at the Menninger Clinic. Meditation activities were conducted either with a magnet suspended over the head, oriented either north-up or south-up, or absent. The effects were evaluated with a questionnaire that assessed five categories: physical, emotional, mental, extrapersonal (psychic), and transpersonal (spiritual). The results were quite amazing, especially with respect to surprising gender differences. When the field was north-up, male subjects tended to be physically and emotionally energized, and females tended to be physically and emotionally inhibited. When the field was south-up, however, the reverse was found—fascinating potential for further exploration.

# Fibromyalgia

The only disorder more prevalent than the common cold is muscle pain. The condition known as fibromyalgia ("fibro" for the soft tissues under the skin, "myo" for muscle, and "algia" for pain) is characterized by varying degrees of discomfort and pain in muscles, ligaments, tendons, and connective tissues throughout the body. Over 90% of patients complain of widespread discomfort or "aching all over." Many also experience fatigue, morning stiffness, sleeping problems, numbness and tingling, headache, irritable bowel syndrome, urinary urgency, anxiety, or depression. It is almost always possible to identify several "trigger points," or areas of unusual tenderness to finger pressure, especially around the neck and shoulders. Although it has been found in adolescents and the elderly, it most often occurs in middle-aged patients, women in the vast majority.

Dr. Rosch notes that about half of the patients link the onset of their symptoms to some sort of stressful event. And stress is even more likely to cause a flare-up of increased pain, fatigue, or tenderness in an already chronic condition.

In chapter 8 we present the promising results of a very recent, as yet unpublished study by Dr. Agatha Colbert on fibromyalgia, as well as a post-polio study: muscle pain and trigger points are features of post-polio syndrome. Post-polio syndrome deals with muscle pain and trigger points. Two doctors who have investigated the use of magnets with this disorder were, like most doctors, very skeptical at first. Drs. Carlos Vallbona and Carlton Hazlewood at Houston's Baylor College of Medicine were both flabbergasted when magnets made their own chronic knee pains disappear in minutes. As they commented, "That was too good to be true."

### Case History: Jean

Jean, a 32-year-old housewife, mother of one child, had been diagnosed with fibromyalgia approximately two years before she came to Dr. Lawrence. She had the classic symptoms of pain, fatigue, and disturbed sleep patterns, plus the eighteen tender points along the body that are considered the hallmark of fibromyalgia.

Following Dr. Lawrence's prescription, Jean slept on a mattress pad embedded with multiple magnets, and felt considerable relief after the first night. After the third night, she had about 70% relief. After four weeks, she estimated 85% relief from her generalized aches and pains involving mostly the back area. Now that she could sleep more restfully, her fatigue levels dropped and normal energy returned. She continues to sleep on the magnetized pad.

## Asthma and Allergies

The action of magnetic fields on asthma works through relaxing spasms of bronchial muscles. It also appears as though the same force will block much of the tendency to spasm.

## Case History: Andrew

Andrew, a 55-year-old man with asthma, had tried all the approaches, especially the broncho-dilators and inhaled steroids, as well as cromolyn. Yet he was still having asthmatic episodes and difficulty breathing. After a cold, the post-nasal drip would set off his bronchial spasms and cause his asthma to get worse. Dr. Lawrence placed magnets over the chest area, and Andrew was able to reduce the use of his dilators and inhalants and breathe more freely.

According to Dr. Lawrence, in New York state, Dr. William Lampard had thirty-three asthmatic patients whom he treated over a period of several years using different types of magnets over the chest area. He measured the forced expiration in a pulmonary function test and found that function was enhanced from 25% to 75% by using magnets. This study included children as well as adults.

However, before reducing medications, asthma patients should check with their physicians. Each case is different.

# Arthritis

The many kinds of arthritis that respond to magnet therapy were discussed in chapter 3, "The Many Faces of Pain." As we noted, arthritis is a condition that cannot be "cured," but the symptoms (chiefly pain) can be alleviated, and mobility regained.

## Case Histories: Marie and Jerry

Marie, a 70-year-old female with aching in her hip and knee, came to Dr. Lawrence with a unique problem: She *had* to be active. She was a grandmother who took care of her four grandchildren. Among her other duties, she had to drive them to school. Even pressing her foot down on the gas or the brakes was a problem for her. He used the magnets over the hip at the side of the greater trochanter and at the front on the inguinal crease. Dr. Lawrence also used the acupuncture points involving the area with the referred pain to the knee. After two days, Marie had 70% relief from pain, just from using the magnets alone.

Jerry, a 26-year-old who played a lot of tennis, was almost a world-class player. Then he developed tennis elbow—pain at the lateral portion of the elbow. Dr. Lawrence used the plasti-form type of magnetic wrap, covering the four areas around the elbow, which is an optimal placement. Jerry wore it when he was playing, except during tournaments because it re-stricted his movement a bit too much. He proclaimed the magnetic wrap a "smashing" success.

## Insomnia and Other Sleep Disorders

Restful sleep is vital to health, to allow the body recuperation time after the day's many stressors. A magnetized mattress pad helps to promote a restful sleep. (Dr. Lawrence uses one him-self.) They aren't inexpensive, but they're worth it. The mus-cle-relaxing effects are only part of the benefit, as you can imagine now that you have learned how magnetism stimulates healing and promotes homeostasis.

Without claiming that it has been validated, here is one foreign report: A double-blind clinical study was done in Japan in 1990 with magnetized mattress pads in three hospitals. The 431 subjects were tested and observed closely for any side effects. The magnetized pads used 104 magnets, each of 750–950-gauss strength. More than 70% of the patients had results within five days. The improvements in back and lower back pain ranged from 68.49 to 92.04%; in lower limb pain from 66.82 to 97.47%; in insomnia from 76.82 to 97.47%; in fatigue from 70.64 to 94.98%. These are remarkable ranges of improvement, and in an amazingly short time. Reportedly there were no side effects. (Source: Dr. Kazuo Shimodair, Tokyo Communications Hospital.) Dr. Rosch cautions, however, that it is not clear what kind of magnets were used, and that the figures might be incorrect.

As he noted in chapter 4, the FDA has recently allowed claims of efficacy of cranioelectrical stimulation for the treatment of anxiety, depression, and insomnia. The low emission therapy (LEET) Symtonic device, which creates a feeble magnetic field in the region of the hypothalamus, has been proven to be a safe and effective treatment for insomnia, based on FDA-designed trials at two leading University Sleep Laboratories. The device was also proven effective for anxiety in similar crossover studies at Harvard Medical School. It has not yet been approved in the U.S. because obtaining FDA approval can be a lengthy and expensive process. The new regulations will hopefully speed up the approval process.

### Case History: Harry

Harry, a 54-year-old male patient of Dr. Lawrence, not only had insomnia and restless sleep, but also "restless legs syndrome." This is when the legs are aching and seem to twitch and move about involuntarily. He had relief and better sleep after his first night of sleeping on a pad with embedded ceramic magnets. He reported he felt much better and more energized in the morning.

# Fatigue

A special form of fatigue—driving fatigue—has responded well to permanent magnet therapy. Bus or truck drivers and long-distance travelers may develop stiff, aching muscles, back pain, or hemorrhoids. Small magnets are embedded in a car-seat cushion for the driver to sit on. Dr. Rosch supplies the following testimonials from users of a magnetized car seat:

Howard Eplin, middle-aged truck driver: "I have found great relief from my tired, aching, lower back pain. Excellent results with a change from barely tolerable, to light, to no pain."

James Canon, long-distance truck driver in Winter Haven, Florida, averaging from 150,000 to 180,000 miles per year: "In December of 1989, I was involved in a truck accident in which I received extensive injuries, including my hip where I now have steel pins holding it in place. You can imagine the pain I have had as I sit in the truck all day going down the highway. I can honestly say that with the magnetic cushion, which I have been using for the last two months, over 90% of my pain has ceased, and I stay fresher, longer while behind the wheel."

Arleigh Nielsen, also a truck driver in Florida: "I have been using the magnetic cushion for two months and I swear by it. Before using the cushion I suffered from bleeding hemorrhoids and back pain—common ailments for long-distance truck drivers. Since using the cushion, my hemorrhoids have all but disappeared and the back pain is gone. As an added benefit, I feel fresh much longer as I'm driving 8 to 10 hours a day. The cushion is a must for truck drivers."

# Back and Spinal Disk Problems

---

Ever since humans came down from the trees and walked upright, we've been having trouble with our backs. In Dr. Lawrence's practice, he has treated thousands of patients with back and disc problems.

### *Case History: Betsy*

Betsy, a housewife in her late thirties, came to Dr. Lawrence in despair. An MRI revealed a 5 mm protrusion of a disk. Surgery had been recommended, but she couldn't afford it because she had four children and a part-time job. Dr. Lawrence gave her a back corset using magnets along the spinal area and over the sacroiliac joints. That, and sleeping on a magnetic pad at night, gave her sufficient relief. Over a period of months, the disk pulled back, which is a natural tendency. Many people go to surgery because the disk is pressing on the nerve and the pain is acute. But if you don't have any serious neurological problems, and you wait long enough, the body causes degeneration of the disk, which pulls back. That's what happened in her case, and within six months she was doing so well she didn't need her magnetic corset as frequently. She continued to sleep on the magnetic mattress.

# Diabetic Neuropathy

---

The numbness, tingling, and pain of peripheral diabetic neuropathy chiefly affects the feet. Dr. Michael Weintraub, Clinical

Professor of Neurology at New York Medical College, did a pilot study using magnetic foot pads on eight patients with diabetes and six with other forms of neuropathy. Six of the diabetic subjects had a reversal or reduction of symptoms (75%), while only three (50%) of the non-diabetic group improved. The study was completed in January 1998, and published in the *American Journal of Pain Management*. The results offer hope for a new way to treat this difficult problem.

# Magnets and Health Around the World

In India, magnetic therapy has been popular for many decades. Magnets are used for helping to clear the arteries and vessels of cholesterol and calcium, for reducing blood pressure, for asthma and bronchitis, migraine headaches, rheumatism, sciatica, and a whole host of other ailments. Permanent magnets are used in various forms, and they have been using magnetized water to improve many health conditions. Perhaps it is related in some way to the "miracle" springs of Europe, such as the one at Lourdes, whose waters have cured so many seekers, but there is no scientific basis for either waters being effective. Unfortunately, this use of magnets on water has not been confirmed in the U.S.

On the other hand, good double-blind studies, as well as good research, has been done in many countries, including Germany, England, France, Spain, Russia, and Eastern Europe on various health problems that yield to magnetic and electromagnetic therapy. Because some studies have not been translated into English, many U.S. scientists are not familiar with this work; but that doesn't mean the work is not valid. The research abroad, especially from India and China, should not be dismissed out of hand. These researchers have blazed a trail. Where magnetic research has been sparse in the U.S., it has been studied extensively throughout the world by prominent and reliable scientists. If we were to limit ourselves only to U.S. research, we would not be fair to our readers.

Dr. Lawrence points out that India has several fine medical schools, including the All-India Institute in Calcutta and the Medical School in Bombay. Granted, most are not up American standards, yet some of the finest scientists in the world today have been trained in India, and the situation regarding the credibility of Indian medical science is rapidly changing. Also in China, medical schools and science have shown a marked upgrade in the last decade. And after all, in these two countries, magnets have been used for thousands of years. Now a closer, more scientific look is being taken in regard to the study of not only electromagnetism, but even more important, the work with static magnets.

American medical authorities have in the past, with justification, declined to accept most of the research done outside the U.S. That situation has changed markedly during the last decade, during which many of the scientists working in other nations actually studied in the U.S. and returned home to continue work. Further, due to the ease of international travel today, foreign scientists meet with American scientists on a regular basis in thousands of conferences throughout the world. The isolation of the past no longer applies. For these reasons, we will mention work done in other countries, particularly research involving static magnets.

As indicated previously, the most impressive research in this area in the last ten years comes to us from other countries, such as Eastern European studies presented by Drs. Pawluk and Markov in chapter 8.

# Homeostasis and Magnetic Deficiency

The body has a point of balance which is called homeostasis. This is a state of health, sometimes referred to as "the steady state." During illness the body is seeking to return to homeostasis—its tendency is to self-heal with its own mechanisms. You could oversimplify and say the body *wants* to be healthy. Illness happens if homeostasis is not maintained when the body is threatened by any stressful challenge. Scientists have thought of homeostasis in terms of chemical and physiological imbalances (blood sugar, calcium, pH, temperature, pressure, heart rate, and so on). We must now also think in terms of *energy* homeostasis.

Dr. Lawrence speculates that an interruption (blockage) or deficiency in the body's electromagnetic energy force is a sign that the body is out of homeostasis. It follows logically that restoring the flow or correcting the deficiency can easily be done by using the same force—that is, magnetic fields.

Dr. K. Nakagawa of Japan has described "magnetic deficiency syndrome" as being the probable cause of many modern illnesses, with stress and fatigue topping the list. He claims we are not spending adequate time in actual contact with the earth, but in high-rise buildings and cars on freeways. We are therefore more deficient in our own magnetic vital force because we are not getting the full benefit of the earth's strong field. (Perhaps that's why we feel better when we walk barefoot on the grass and spend a lot of time in Nature away from the city.) A further problem may compound this syndrome: Some scientists claim the earth's own magnetic field is diminishing, is far less strong than it was in the days of our cave ancestors.

*Whatever the cause, it is becoming clear that the preservation and balance of magnetic energy in the body may be possible with the help of permanent magnets.*

## Let Nature Be Your Healer

Nature has always been the source of healing medicines, while medical theories and practices come and go. In this chapter you have seen that magnetic therapy has a wide range of applications, and there are even more possibilities out there. Whatever your health problem(s) might be, it is worth considering whether a basic force of Nature, such as magnetism, might be a good option.

> *Let Nature be your teacher.*
> *Spontaneous wisdom breathed by health.*
> —William Wordsworth

# CHAPTER 7

# The Safety of Permanent Magnet Therapy

| • Resonance | • Extremely Low Frequency Fields |
|---|---|

P hysicians using permanent magnets or static magnetic fields for the first time are often surprised at how rapidly they bring about improvements, and are pleased at the lack of side effects. As mentioned in the last chapter, Drs. Carlos Vallbona and Carlton Hazlewood wrote about their trial with post-polio patients: "The fact that none of our patients reported any discomfort resulting from the use of magnetic devices and that no complications have been reported in the literature supports the notion that low-intensity magnetic fields produced by permanent magnets or electromagnetic devices are biologically safe." (*Archives of Physical Medicine and Rehabilitation* Vol. 78, Nov. 1997.)

Potential side effects of permanent magnets are minimal, and not harmful, as many studies have shown. Magnets appear to be an ideal form of therapy, since they will either help you or not; and if they do not, will not cause serious harm. However, we should look at all sides of the issue. We would not want to make a sweeping claim that magnetic therapy is totally harmless.

The following warnings for use of therapeutic magnets have been raised: for patients who are pregnant, and for those who have pacemakers or use electrical diffusion devices. Such patients are advised to consult their physicians.

The matter of adaptation should be remembered. The body's cells tend to adapt, so that the effect is weakened. Magnets work best if not left on twenty-four hours a day, or for days at a time, but when worn in cycles. Dr. Rosch agrees that if magnets take away your pain, you should experiment by removing them to see how long your relief lasts. On the other hand, he points out that it may often take days or even weeks to note an effect. For example, in the diabetic neuropathy study referred to in the previous chapter, patients had magnets applied twenty-four hours a day for four months, and it took over a month for some patients to achieve benefits.

# Resonance

The use of strong magnetic fields in diagnosis (MRIs, or magnetic resonance imaging) has been in existence for twenty years or more. The work of government licensing agencies and health agencies such as NIH (National Institutes of Health) has shown that the MRI's strong magnetic fields have no harmful effects. These fields run up to as many as 15 tesla, which is approximately 150,000 to 200,000 gauss. The MRI is considered a safe procedure for everyone, although a caveat is given that patients will not be allowed to have the MRI if they have any metal in their bodies or are using a pacemaker. However, recent work has shown that even those with pacemakers or metallic parts in their bodies can safely undergo MRI if the procedure is done in proper fashion.

Also, professionals recommend that pregnant women not undergo MRIs, but this is based mostly on the prevailing rationale of the medical profession regarding pregnant women, which includes precaution against drugs and anything unnecessary or off the beaten path—no matter how safe. In general, this is a wise policy. Dr. Abe Liboff, a physicist at Oakland University in Rochester, Michigan, did some observations of MRIs along with people who were exposed every day. He concluded that there was no indication that even very large fields cause damage.

MRIs are superior to x-rays for providing a picture of what is going on inside the brain and body. The technique was originally called "nuclear magnetic resonance" since this is the property that makes the procedure so valuable. The term "nuclear" was dropped to avoid scaring patients, since it is linked in everyone's mind to nuclear war and atomic bombs. An interesting note: MRI might well be more effective than mammography in screening women for breast cancer, since it is a three-dimensional rather than two-dimensional image. However, the cost is prohibitive at this time.

# Extremely Low Frequency Fields

Now we must deal with an issue you have no doubt heard about—the possible dangers of electromagnetic "pollution." There has been talk that harmful effects, even certain forms of cancer, are promoted by such things as power lines, radio transmitters, home appliances, electric blankets, and computers. This thought may have lurked at the back of your mind like a dark shadow since you started this book.

Our world abounds in paradoxes, in two-edged swords. Oxygen is a prime example—we need it to survive, yet the normal processes of oxidation in the body can damage our cells. Electromagnetism is also a two-edged sword, with potential for both healing and damage, depending on its form.

It is true that by surrounding ourselves with too many *low-frequency* electromagnetic fields (ELFs) for a significant time, we become subject to physiological damage by long-term exposure. The conflicting, overlapping fields, however weak they may be, cumulatively interfere with our normal biology. This bombardment of ELFs from man-made devices represents the opposite side of the sword from the healing side. In addition, the benefits of technology expose us to radiation—a kind of radiation earth's inhabitants have never experienced before.

Dr. Lawrence explains: Any electrically charged conductor generates two types of invisible fields, electrical and magnetic, which are called electromagnetic fields when combined. The electromagnetic spectrum has a high end and a low in regard to frequency and energy. The high energy end consists of short wavelength forms of radiation called ionizing radiation. X-rays, for example, are at the high end and produce ionizing radiation that can be dangerous if not properly used.

At the other end of the spectrum are the longer wave-length waves where we find the extremely low frequency ELF waves, which are generally not considered dangerous at this point in research. Although much money is being spent at this time for research on ELF waves, researchers have not yet demonstrated firm conclusions regarding potential harm. However, some eminent scientists feel there may be harmful, difficult-to-find side effects that bear watching.

Fields generated by TV, video players, and other common electrical apparatus we all use do produce ELF waves. These ELFs involve alternating current or pulsed direct current at frequencies (60 cycles per second) that do not resonate with the natural human frequencies (12 cycles per second). But they do not produce the dramatic effects on the human body as do the higher frequency wave fields such as those of x-rays. All electrical conductors such as common home wiring generate magnetic fields, albeit low-energy ones, and these apparently cause little if any harmful biological changes.

The existence of this dark shadow should not discourage the reader from investigating the benefits of magnetic therapy. Magnets, as we have stated before, are safe for use in therapy—far safer than most drugs. Still, it is always advisable to be sure the person applying the magnets is experienced and highly trained in the therapy. However, *electro*magnetic "damage" is not something that will result from permanent magnet therapy.

Dr. Robert Becker, the same orthopedist who pioneered electromagnetic therapy for bone fracture healing, has written *Cross Currents,* an excellent book on the subject of ELF pollution. The average consumer might find this helpful to remember: There is a world of difference between the blizzard of weak magnetic fields in the environment, whether indoors or out, and the healing magnetic field coming from the permanent magnet taped to the skin of one's aching arm.

In *Cross Currents,* Dr. Becker writes about the problem of effects from microwaves, radio waves, and electric or magnetic fields: "Today's environment is a latticework of crisscrossing signals in which there's always the possibility of synergistic effects or the "construction" of new ELF signals from the patterns of interference between two higher frequencies."

Ross Adey, Professor of Biochemistry at University of California, Riverside, puts it this way: "We are bathed in a veritable sea of man-made electromagnetic fields, the likes of which have never existed in the whole history of earth's biological evolution. Not that it is inherently harmful, but viewed objectively, it is very difficult to prove safe." Professor Adey has been writing about and experimenting in this field for the last twenty-five years. He notes that if we are to make progress in understanding the potential health risks of ELFs, we must take into account the rapidly changing engineering technologies. Older FM (frequency modulation) systems are switching to digital transmission that, in essence, expose the user to a microwave field that pulses at low rates. Professor Adey explains: "This appears to greatly increase occurrence of a wide range of physiological interactions, particularly in the brain and immune system, *not seen in the older FM systems,* where the radio signal does not vary in intensity throughout the transmission."

In regard to concerns you might have that damage from power lines and magnetic therapy might be related, James Souder, who designs magnetic devices, explains it clearly: "Electromagnetic fields surrounding power lines are generated by alternating currents which produce a pulsing field having both a magnetic component and a separate and distinct electric field component." Permanent magnets produce static or motionless fields that are quite different. There is no electrical component and there are no health hazards.

So please remember, when we discuss magnets used in therapy, we are talking about magnetic fields, not electrical fields. Since the issue of safety is not, at this time, a concern for those being treated with static or permanent magnets, we won't belabor the point. We should mention that if you are being treated with electromagnetic apparatus, ask the manufacturer about safe usage. Manufacturers of electromagnetic equipment are constrained to supply this information to the consumer anyway.

To summarize, permanent or static magnets have definitely been shown not to produce dangerous biological effects. Dangers of ELF wave generation, which do not involve permanent magnets, are being studied (60 Hertz fields for example). Presently, these are also considered not to be harmful. But research continues and the final vote is not yet in.

Ideally, we would like current research on the potential hazards of ELF pollution to build bridges that will lead us to a point in the future when medical science can use *magnetic* therapy to counter any harmful effects of *electro*magnetic pollution.

The reason, dear reader, this chapter is so short is that we are convinced the magnetic fields from permanent magnets used to relieve pain and promote healing are extremely safe.

# CHAPTER 8

# Twenty-First Century Medicine

## *Late-Breaking News*

- First World Congress on Magnetotherapy and the Congress on Stress
- North American Academy of Magnetic Therapy Conference
- ADD Children
- Physicists, Doctors, and Dreamers
- Headaches
- An Important Beginning: Study on Fibromyalgia
- The Skeptic
- Referred Pain
- Magnet Design

New developments are fast unfolding as the excitement spreads about the many-faceted applications and benefits of magnetic therapy. One of the best ways for an emerging therapy to find footing and begin growing toward acceptance is through a conference—all those interested come together for a few days to present their ideas, answer questions, and then spend time together over meals or in hallways exchanging views, arguing finer points, and sparking each other in new directions.

# First World Congress on Magnetotherapy and the Congress on Stress

The growing interest in magnetic therapies is vividly illustrated by the phenomenal increase in worldwide conferences devoted to this subject in the past two years. The First World Congress on Magnetotherapy in London was organized by Roger Coghill. A host of new magnetic therapies were presented from England, Europe, and Eastern Europe that were unknown in the United States.

The 1997 Congress on Stress in Montreux, Switzerland, included some new magnetic therapies and also featured Dr. Demetrio Sodi-Pallares, who showed x-rays of patients with advanced metastatic bone cancer and terminal heart disease not responsive to any treatment. These patients were now perfectly healthy a year or so later with his combined nutritional and electromagnetic approach. As indicated in chapter 10, it seems quite possible that nutritional interventions can enhance permanent magnet therapy, at least in fibromyalgia.

Dr. Saul Liss had shown at a prior Stress Congress that cranioelectrical stimulation could significantly increase serotonin and endorphin levels, which might explain its efficacy for depression and pain relief. At this meeting, he demonstrated that one brand of permanent magnets could increase endorphins 45% in an hour or two. Could this be why putting a magnet on one part of the body can relieve pain at a distant site that has nothing to do with acupuncture meridians?

Dr. Rosch chaired a conference organized by Dr. Norman Shealy in Branson, Missouri, a few months later to celebrate "The First Thirty Years of Modern Electrotherapy." The *Electreat* spark gap stimulator was patented back in 1917, but many years later it was still the first device Dr. Shealy used to treat pain. He was so impressed with the potential that he gave up neurosurgery and has spent the last 30 years trying to improve pain therapy without drugs. He started with the first TENS device, teamed up with Dr. Saul Liss, and their association has now culminated in the She-Li TENS and GigaTENS instrumentation. Magnets were discussed at this meeting, as well as one conducted by the Bioelectromagnetic Society (BEMS) in April 1997 in Bologna, Italy, to honor Galvani's getting the ball rolling. It was arranged by Dr. Martin Blank, president of BEMS, who told Dr. Rosch that in past years, most presentations had dealt with basic science, and that he was amazed that this year, clinical studies were in the majority. Dr. Rosch also reported on a study by Dr. Michael Weintraub that appeared the previous week, showing that magnetic insoles relieved pain and other symptoms in three out of four patients with diabetic neuropathy.

(By the way: BEMS is one of the most prominent of these organizations, and applicants for membership are carefully screened. Other organizations with magnetism in their title have sprung up, but these are open to anyone, and it is possible that their publications could be self-serving if funding comes from a source that has a vested financial interest. One of the reasons for writing this book is that the authors felt strongly that much of the information about magnets in existing books and articles is misleading and inaccurate.)

Magnets were also the topic of discussion at the November 1997 meeting held in Bloomington, Minnesota, by Dr. Bjorn Nordenstrom's Biologically Closed Electrical Circuit (BCEC) organization. In addition to Chinese physicians reporting on cancer cures using the Nordenstrom technique mentioned in chapter 4, there were fascinating presentations showing how electrotherapy could improve senile macular degeneration and glaucoma, and stating that similar results had been obtained with magnets. Dr. Rosch is now involved in double-blind studies for both of these conditions as well as for diabetic neuropathy. During this conference, Dr. Nordenstrom said that he thought the energy flowing in his "electrical circulatory system was probably the same as *Qi (chi)*, but nobody knows what *Qi* is."

# North American Academy
# of Magnetic Therapy Conference

Now the latest: The 1998 conference of the North American Academy of Magnetic Therapy was held in Los Angeles, California, at the Furama Hotel, only a few minutes by taxi from the Los Angeles International Airport. Physicians, physicists, physical therapists, and designers of magnetic devices made an interesting if sometimes volatile mix. One hopeful sign for the future was that the American Medical Association sent a physician representative.

There was healthy controversy over the major question: "How?" Exactly and by what mechanisms do the magnetic fields work their healing wonders? This is the thrust of science: Find the how, measure the results, and repeat the experiment to prove it valid. Or, to put it another way: You've got to find the mechanism or people can't believe it.

Here are some conference high points, which do not necessarily give fair coverage to each individual presenter, nor present all details, due to major constraints of time. And some presentations delved so deeply into the esoteric depths of physics as to fall outside the parameters of this book.

Dr. Lawrence opened the meeting by stating that magnet therapy stands today where acupuncture once did, when the practice looked as though it might never be accepted in the U.S. However, this 1998 Academy meeting had the support of the Los Angeles County Medical Association, an important first. Magnets, said Dr. Lawrence, help as much or more than any drug. "I envision the day when magnets will be part of standard medical practice. I am an optimist, but not a fool. I sincerely believe magnet therapy cannot be stopped, but will take its place as a valid therapeutic approach to many problems, especially pain."

Dr. Lawrence continued: It should be noted a lot of pioneering work was done with animals, and animals don't lie (nor are they subject to the placebo effect). Permanent magnets are helping horses—$3.5 to $4 million worth of magnets were sold to horse owners last year. At Santa Anita racetrack, 50% of horses had magnets applied. The race horse is an easy followup—it has to run better and win races. At the racetrack, you know when something works. There is no mysticism to it. But magnets also work on the physiology of the human body. "There is a great deal of science leading into what we are doing," he concluded, "doing what we can for the illnesses that flesh is heir to, finding how magnets can be applied."

Dr. C. K. Chou of the City of Hope Medical Center in Duarte, California, made the first presentation with his review of work being done in China with electrical current and localized cancer tumors. (This important work, based on Dr. Bjorn Nordenstrom's theories of the body's electrical system mentioned previously, is described in chapter 11.)

The next speaker, William Pawluk, M.D., summarized the exciting results of 343 studies done on magnetic therapy in Eastern Europe. One of the chief sources was the Institute of Magnetic Therapy in the Czech Republic, and other studies were from Hungary and Russia. This was the new data the attendees were hoping to get; there was only an unspoken sense of disappointment that it was not from the United States.

The results Dr. Pawluk cited were truly impressive, covering an amazing range, a whole spectrum of conditions: leg phlebitis (blood clot), cerebral atherosclerosis, cervical arthritis, bronchitis, and polyneuritis in children. One of the studies dealt with pancreatitis, a condition for which there is very little treatment. Checkerboard, flexible magnetic pads were used, first on animals, then on eighty humans. There were no controls in this study. The magnets covered subjects' abdomen and gastric area and/or the lumbar region of the back. After twenty-one days, "significant benefits" and clinical improvement resulted.

Magnetic fields helped heal post-radiation tissue damage, and the post-operative healing of gliomas. Rheumatoid arthritis patients were helped by magnetic therapy. All improved, although some took a downturn first. Dr. Pawluk noted that very severe cases of rheumatoid arthritis were not likely to benefit. Complicated bone fractures, however, showed significant improvement through recovery of circulation. Swelling and pain decreased, and rehabilitation time was shortened. A study using static magnetic fields on burn patients demonstrated reduction in pain, faster healing, and 232 patients with amputated limbs also fared better with their phantom pain problems. Chronic prostatitis patients showed dramatic pain improvement, as did those with corneal trauma, retinitis pigmentosa, endometriosis, carpal tunnel syndrome, psychological instability—an impressive list. Dr. Pawluk also summarized the major magnetic effects found in these studies as: vasodilation, analgesia, anti-inflammatory, spasmolytic, anti-edema (swelling), and healing acceleration.

Dr. Pawluk concluded on the hopeful note that, although no similar studies have been done in the U.S. as yet, "all of us here will be part of that."

# ADD Children

One of the conference high points came next, via a calm, almost understated report from a doctor in clinical pediatric practice, Dr. Bernard Margolis of Harrisburg, Pennsylvania. He opened by saying he is a clinician, not research-oriented. But what he then described cast a hush over the room of M.D.s, Ph.D.s, and D.O.s. He treated his young patients with static magnets for asthma, burns, sports injuries, and, most importantly, for ADD (Attention Deficit Disorder), which is also sometimes called ADHD (Attention Deficit Hyperactive Disorder).

ADD, widespread among America's children, has been called "the disease of the year." The symptoms include difficulty reading, inability to stay focused or concentrated, hyperactive, restless, impulsive behavior. Schools send thousands of these kids to doctors' offices. The common response from physicians has been a medication, chiefly Ritalin, a psycho-stimulant that paradoxically can have calming influence on such children.

The problem is the side effects of depressed appetite and therefore slower growth, disturbed sleep patterns, and other emotional problems such as aggression and depression.

When Dr. Margolis first heard about magnet therapy, he thought it was totally off the wall. However, he decided to try it a few times. He treated a four-year-old with bad burns on both hands from a fall onto Grandma's wood stove. The hand treated with magnets, in contrast to the other hand (both dressed with bandages), had no edema or blistering. In a dramatic episode, a girl with asthma was having severe problems in spite of steroid inhalers and antibiotics. Dr. Margolis offered the mother the choice of trying the magnets to reduce the asthma or taking the child to the hospital. The mother agreed to try magnets. Dr. Margolis taped small magnets of 700 gauss to the girl's chest. In two hours all signs of respiratory difficulty were gone. The next morning she woke up well.

Now sold on the efficacy of magnets, Dr. Margolis set up a case study for ADD. This was a simple case study, without controls or placebos. He convened the parents in his office one evening at the beginning of summer and asked their permission. He explained the safety of magnets. To his surprise, every single parent was willing. He took some of the young patients off their medications, in order to check results against those on none, some, or a lot. He started with thirty, and two dropped out because they didn't want to wear or use the products. Ages were from five to eighteen, and all but two patients were male.

Dr. Margolis used static magnets of different kinds, some placed on the chest, some insoles in shoes, some sleep pads. They were to return the products at the end of the week, at the time the parents mailed back reports. Nineteen of the twenty-eight had significant improvements in the first week, judged by the best judges in this case—parents. By far the most telling comment was from one mother who happens to hold a Ph.D.: "It was like night and day with him. He was lovable with magnets, and without, he was up for adoption."

In another case, a sibling was offered use of the magnet sleep pad for one night and refused. She said: "I'd love to have it, but please, don't ever take it off his bed."

All of the nine who did not respond only used one magnet product. Now Dr. Margolis recommends using the magnetic sleep pad at night and insoles during the day, both for the surrounding coverage and for easier compliance. Most of the children didn't like the possibility of being set apart as different or having the task of placing the magnet on the chest area. With the magnetic sleep pads, they did not wake up as early and were not as agitated and difficult to cope with in getting ready for the day.

Dr. Margolis noted that ADD is pervasive in our society, not so much in other cultures. He cautioned that magnets alone cannot do everything. Nutrition and other factors are vital, and many of the children have self-esteem problems. The goal, however, is to get them off the psycho-stimulants. He appealed to other professionals to help seek these answers: How long can the good effects of magnets last before the children revert to their previous condition? Should lower or higher strength magnetic fields be used? Should the therapy include intervals when magnets are not used? "Researchers, please try to get a handle on this."

Dr. Marko Markov, a distinguised physicist and authority on the psycho-physiological effects of magnetic fields, rose to his feet and thanked Dr. Margolis for being a pioneer in this gray area, an area where no one else has ventured.

This case study, by the way, is being submitted for publication. Details on it and other advances can be obtained by contacting Dr. Lawrence or Dr. Rosch (see chapter 11).

## Physicists, Doctors, and Dreamers

Dr. Abe Liboff, another distinguished pioneer in the field, re-emphasized that there is no such thing as a "unipolar" or single pole magnet. It is possible to have a "positive" or "negative" electrical charge, but not a positive or negative magnetic field.

Dr. Liboff stated that the simplicity of magnets belies their complexity. It's not like adding a pinch of something as in a prescription. Pharmaceuticals have only two variables: dose and formulation. A magnetic field also has dose (intensity), but, because of its vector nature, one also has to consider spatial factors (for example, gradient).

New materials for magnets give options not available thirty or forty years ago. Dr. Liboff's prediction for the future: Because magnetic fields interact with living systems, and because they are noninvasive, and because they are beautifully complex, magnetic therapy holds an incredible potential for exquisite fine-tuning in patient treatment.

Betty Sisken, Ph.D., Professor at the Center for Biomedical Engineering at the University of Kentucky, is also the incoming president of the Bioelectromagnetic Society, the most prestigious organization in this field. She spoke about pulsed magnetic fields for nerve regeneration in both animal and in vitro studies. After crash injuries, using various chemical agents and pulsed magnetic fields, the nerve growth factor was induced and the nerve cells began to regenerate quickly, approximately 20–25% above that of normal.

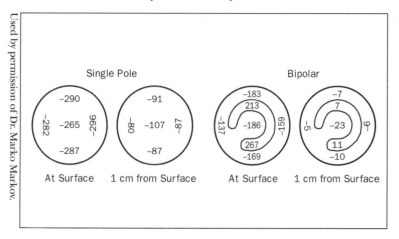

**Figure 8.1**

Gauss Ratings of a Single Pole of a Magnet
and a Bipolar Configuraion

On day two of the meeting, Dr. Rosch began with an overview of the history of electromagnetic therapy, and urged an open mind to effects that can't always be explained. What we need to know is how magnets can be improved, how to help more people, he said. We don't always have satisfactory explanations. Look at faith healing. It does occur, but science can't explain it. Kirlian photography shows the "spiritual" aura of a person recorded on film. Dr. Rosch has a study showing that a healer could cause a surge of 100 volts in the EEG of a shielded individual 15 feet away. Scientists shouldn't dismiss something because they can't explain why it is so.

Static magnetic fields versus moving? Precise placement of permanent magnets at acupuncture points may seem at odds with the good results from the magnetic mattresses and sleep pads. Both have value.

Theories don't have to be correct. Only facts do. And the facts are that magnetic therapy can provide a wide range of clinical benefits. Recent studies confirm that permanent magnets can and do relieve pain in a variety of situations, but a lot of research still needs to be done. Who will do it? There's the rub. There is no big money in such research, no way to protect it. Dr. Rosch gave examples of how electromagnetic therapies had been surprisingly effective in metastatic cancer, advanced heart disease, multiple sclerosis, diabetes, osteoporosis, Parkinson's disease, and insomnia.

Dr. Rosch also reported on a new form of electronic stimulation for depression called rTMS (repetitive transcranial magnetic stimulation). Drs. Shealy and Liss had previously shown that cranioelectrical stimulation using electrodes on both sides of the scalp were a safe and effective treatment for depression, and raised serotonin levels just like Prozac, but did it quicker and without any side effects. This new approach uses a hand-held device aimed at a specific area of the brain shown to have an energy disturbance. It is safe and painless, producing quick results in patients resistant to drug therapy.

"We are dreamers of magnetic therapy," stated Marko Markov, Ph.D. Dr. Markov has done twenty years of research on magnets, mostly in Bulgaria, and has extensive knowledge of Eastern European and Russian research. He noted that the meeting represented an enormous acceleration of interest and scientific improvement in the area of research and development, opening new frontiers in biology and medicine. He stressed it is very important that dedicated scientists are entering the area of magnetic therapy, in order to plant it in the U.S. on a serious basis.

Magnet therapy is able to treat the source of disease, rather than only the symptoms. While $60 million has been spent on research on the harmful effects of electromagnetic fields, almost nothing has been granted for magnet therapy.

But times are changing, due to the rapid increase of public and media interest. The media, however, tend to indicate that the use of magnets is quackery, which creates a bad atmosphere, and the medical profession in the U .S. has not been prepared to accept it. The research that began in Russia in 1977 covered fifty various diseases and conditions. So "new" technology in the U.S. may be old news to Europe.

For example, Dr. R. Kikut of Latvia in 1975 treated 1,000 patients with 2,000 gauss magnets for brain aneurysms. No further strokes were reported. In Hungary, Dr. A. Guseo used low-frequency ELF magnetic fields for multiple sclerosis. There was work done between 1992 and 1996 on "electrochemotherapy" of cancer patients, to help make more efficient pathways for the intravenous drips.

As to the question of which is more important, the electro or magnetic component, it is best to look at all the possible mechanisms in the systems and the cells. The cell membrane is a powerful amplifier, acts as an ion pump, and has effects on enzymes. The calcium ion in particular is a key player for interactions.

Dr. Markov told of his work, which showed a marked drop-off in magnetic field strength one centimeter from the skin with bipolar magnets. This was not as pronounced with monopolar magnets. (see figure 8.1).

"The goal is to complete our dreams," he said, and ended his talk with: "We are here to learn."

# Headaches

Dr. Joseph Kleinkort, a physical therapist from Arlington, Texas, touched a shared truth when he observed how hard it is to make a good decision until all information is gathered—a clinician's point of view. But what if you are a sick person? Dr. Kleinkort had set up a chronic pain clinic for the Air Force, had worked under Dr. Paul Nogier, the father of auricular acupuncture, and had learned acupuncture from him.

Headaches strike 66% of the population, he noted. Some are related to depression, fatigue, or structures of the cervical spine. He recorded the progress of 2,000 patients with cervical and jaw changes. These are difficult to treat, but can greatly be modulated even with static magnets. He feels that neodymium magnets are very beneficial to stimulate the correct acupuncture points, and he thinks they can significantly alter the flow of *chi.*

For some people, he found wearing the magnets twenty-four hours a day was not good, for others, very preventive. He treated migraine and sinus headaches as well. But he pointed out that more research is critical. It is fortunate, he said, that a number of the big manufacturing companies are considering funding research studies, "proper" studies with double-blind and placebo controls.

Another physical therapist, Raymond Cralle of Delray Beach, Florida, reported on success with magnet therapy in tennis elbow. He also showed slides of a spastic child helped by a magnetic mattress. Like the ADD children, this child would wake up rested, having slept well. The mattress even helped quadriplegics breathe better and sleep through the night.

At this point, Dr. Marko Markov returned to show amazing color slides of post-operative healing from plastic surgery, which came from Dr. Daniel Man of Boca Raton, Florida. When a magnet was applied to a hematoma, the difference was visible in forty-eight hours. Ecchymosis (black and blue bruising) from liposuction treated for twenty-four hours with a magnetic pad cleared nearly the whole area where applied (see figure 8.2).

Dr. Markov also showed a dramatic picture of an amputated hand that was replaced in surgery, during which surgeons tried to reconnect the blood vessels. A range of 1,000-gauss magnets were placed on the surface. In five weeks the hand had completely healed (for another example of a magnet's healing power on a hand, see figure 8.3).

Dr. Markov noted that perhaps "magnetic field strength" would be a better term to use than gauss strength. He emphasized that the *depth* of penetration is what's important.

# An Important Beginning:
## Study on Fibromyalgia

Dr. Agatha Colbert from Newton Center, Massachusetts, and affiliated with Tufts University, gave the first report of a just completed study on the effect of magnetic mattresses on fibromyalgia. This is a mysterious pain condition with no clear cause that hits seven times more women than men. Most patients go from doctor to doctor, and take test after test, before even getting the correct diagnosis. Then there is the problem of getting relief. The list of symptoms is a long one, headed by pains and rigid muscles, and often including stiffness, migraine headache, trouble sleeping, pervasive fatigue, depression, and gastric disorders. There are several tender "points." Neurotransmitters are involved in fibromyalgia, and as you have learned, nerves transmit pain signals. The requirements to confirm the diagnosis, as Dr. Colbert noted, are chronic pain present for longer than three months, both above and below the waist, and at least eighteen tender or trigger points.

To date there are no satisfactory treatments, though trials have been done on drugs. Psychotropics, though not significantly helpful, are still prescribed. Perhaps one-third respond to Elavil, but with hangover-like side effects. Valium and anti-inflammatories show no lasting relief at all. With biofeedback, there can be 30–40% improvement, and some 70% will have a better pain threshold with acupuncture. Daily relaxation and self-hypnosis help some.

In the test started in March 1997, approved by Tufts Medical School, the question was: Does sleeping on magnetic mattresses influence the pain and sleep disturbances seen in fibromyalgia? The thirty subjects were not allowed any medications or other new treatments during the study. The doctors in the study didn't know which mattresses (some had no magnets) went to which patients. Using a questionnaire, the patients marked the changes in their symptoms, the number of tender points, and so on. The point count in the magnetic group went way down, other pain symptoms went down, and the sleep pattern improved. The functional ability was not that significantly changed.

The patients also kept a daily record and were able to call in twenty-four hours a day. A biostatistician on the project who works for the NIH was extremely skeptical in the beginning, then stated that the statistical differences in pain and sleep left no doubt.

The patients who had the sham mattresses were given an opportunity to try the real ones, and a month or two later all

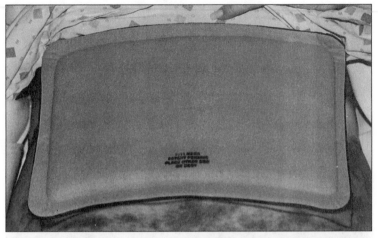

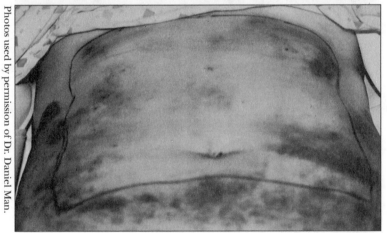

**Figure 8.2**

patients were given the opportunity to buy the mattresses or return them. All the sham mattresses were sent back, but all the magnetic mattresses except one were purchased by the patients.

The chief skeptic at the meeting, Dr. Josyh Kirschvink, found it impossible to believe it was a properly blinded study,

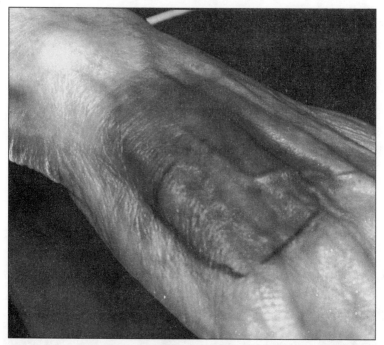

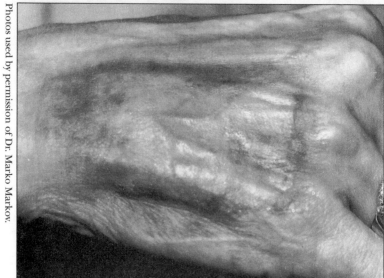

Photos used by permission of Dr. Marko Markov.

**Figure 8.3**

that the patients didn't know which mattresses had magnets. Not good science, he said.

Dr. Colbert explained the patients had informed consent, were told they might get the real mattresses or they might not. The important factor is that these were patients for whom nothing else had worked, and all were helped.

# The Skeptic

Then came the skeptic's turn to speak. Josyh Kirschvink, Ph.D., a professor at the California Institute of Technology, was surprised to have been invited to the conference in the first place. Dr. Lawrence, however, rightly felt that controversy would be stimulating and productive.

Dr. Kirschvink expressed doubts whether magnets have a therapeutic effect in humans. He emphasized the need for more double-blind studies, an opinion which all essentially shared.

In 1992 Dr. Kirschvink, a geologist, and his associates at Cal Tech had discovered magnetite, the same type as is found in lodestones, in human brain tissue. Now he talked about magnetite found in birds, bees, and fish, and how this substance is believed to aid them in navigation. He then went into very technical exposition of his continuing work with magnetite in the biological sphere. His comments regarding potential dangers of magnetic therapy, as well as the importance of true double-blind studies, stimulated some very lively discussion, especially among the physicists. Participants generally felt that, instead of more theories being postulated, more scientific facts were needed. As Dr. Kirschvink pointed out, this was a "heated agreement." Everyone was in harmony on one point: More money should be allotted by our government in grants for specific research on magnetic therapy.

# Referred Pain

Carlton Hazlewood, Ph.D., a physiologist affiliated with Baylor College of Medicine in Houston, Texas, presented an important case study of post-polio syndrome which occurs in a small percentage of polio victims twenty to thirty years after initial attack. He pointed out that this is a nonrecurring population, which may be one reason drug companies are not interested. Post-polio patients have increased sensitivity to stimuli and receptivity to pain. Typically, their pain is myofascial (muscles of the face) or arthritic. He found that placing a magnet on a trigger point usually relieved referred pain. He added that sometimes, after a point has been identified and treated, another point will surface elsewhere.

Dr. Hazlewood said that as a physiologist, he particularly notices facial expressions. A typical patient was a woman suffering from migraines who couldn't move her head or smile, but one could see the pain in her eyes. Migraine sufferers often describe the pain as feeling like the skull is about to fly off. Magnets of various configurations were used to wipe out the migraine.

Another patient with wrist pain couldn't open a door. A magnet was placed on the trigger point, and brought pain relief. That was three years ago, and since then the patient developed pain in other areas, but not the wrist. Dr. Hazlewood noted that mobility was of crucial importance to these patients, adding greatly to their sense of well-being.

What led up to these observations is of interest, too. Earlier in 1997, Dr. Hazlewood had joined in a study also on post-polio syndrome with Carlos Vallbona, M.D., at Baylor University. (The results were published in the *American Journal of Pain Management,* November 1997.) Dr. Vallbona, at first skeptical himself, conducted a rigorous study that in turn was built on much earlier observations, including a study from Sweden in 1938 that showed that electromagnetic fields relieved sciatica and arthralgia.

The results of the published 1997 study with Dr. Vallbona were surprising. One patient was a priest whose post-polio symptoms, especially back pain, made his celebrating of Mass very difficult. A few minutes of application with a magnetic field and the pain was gone. The priest pronounced it a miracle.

Fifty volunteers were tested, some receiving a sham magnet as controls. The twenty-nine who received an active magnet reported, on a pain scale of 0 to 10 (worst), a reduction from 9.6 to 4.4. Those who received the sham magnets had a smaller decline, from 9.5 to 8.4.

# Magnet Design

The polar controversy was mentioned by James Souder, a designer of magnetic devices. The unipole, he explained, only means the orientation of north or south to the body. What is important in the therapy is *depth* or penetration. So is motion. The moving of the field helps to explain a great deal. However, the observations about north and south, positive and negative, should not be written off.

The really significant thing magnets accomplish, in his view, is muscle relaxation. Magnets will stop muscle spasm, stop the contraction. For instance, on a long car drive, the muscles tend to shorten, fibers overlap. But if you use a magnetic car seat, this won't happen. He noted the success of magnets in fibromyalgia patients, to stop a muscle contraction, a pain flare.

There was far more to this meeting. Other speakers included Arthur Pilla, Ph.D., from Mount Sinai Hospital and Medical School in New York, on the physics aspect of static magnetic fields, and Richard Luben, Ph.D., on electromagnetic bone healing.

By now the reader has much to consider and absorb. The coming together of minds at the Furama Hotel—of M.D.s, Ph.D.s, D.O.s, physical therapists, magnet manufacturers, and interested others—brought a blend of hope and caution, disagreement and dreams, hard science and hasty science, long medical terms and an occasional reference to spirit and God.

Conference participants noted that millions of people in India, China, Japan, and Eastern Europe have used magnets, and no questions have arisen of any dangers. But people do worry about the possibilities; therefore more research, more studies, more statistics are needed. Everyone is greatly looking forward to next year's conference. Meanwhile, the public can take advantage of these steps to bring magnetic therapy forward.

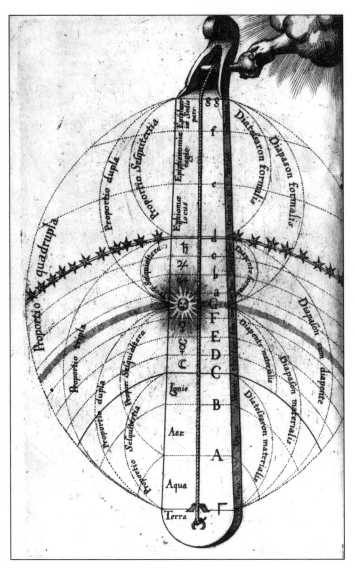

Pictured here is the Cosmic Monochord according to Robert
Fludd: God turns the tuning peg, to achieve harmony in all the
universe from the heavens down to earth. (Reproduced with
permission from the Department of Printing and Graphic Arts,
The Houghton Library, Harvard University.)

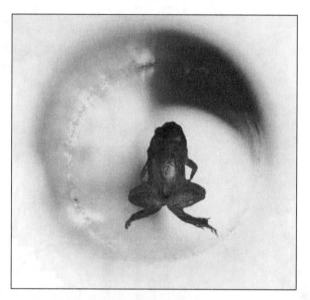

Researchers from the Nijmegen High Field Magnet Laboratory in The Netherlands levitated a living frog in a magnetic field of 160,000 gauss as shown here. For more on levitating objects with magnets, see pages 202–203. (Photo used by permission of the University of Nijmegen, Dr. Andrey Gein.)

# CHAPTER 9

# The Skeptics

| • Placebos | • Further Sources of Skepticism |

*The exploration of the atomic and subatomic world in the twentieth century has revealed an unexpected limitation of classical ideas, and has necessitated a radical revision of many of our basic concepts.*

—Fritjof Capra

Skepticism definitely has its place. It is important to question every new medical therapy and medication that comes along, because the health of millions could be affected. Those millions rely on the expertise and experience of physicians. As Dr. Stephen J. Gould, president-elect of the American Association for the Advancement of Science, has written in *Science* (1998; 279:812–813): "Human choice, not the intrinsic content of science, determines the outcome—and scientists, as human beings, therefore have a special responsibility to provide counsel rooted in expertise."

Dr. Lawrence and Dr. Rosch, feeling this responsibility as they do, wish to allow skeptics their say. This provides a kind of professional homeostasis, if you will, a balance of openness and caution. Good science and good controversy go together.

Outside the field are those who have no faith at all in magnet therapy; they too deserve to be heard. Skepticism is a long tradition—its origin is the early Greek philosophers. The main proponent was named Arcesilaus, who founded "academic skepticism" in the Platonic Academy around 250 B.C. He and his followers believed that reason could be found on every side of the question, so philosophic agreement should always be withheld. Therefore, it was impossible to attain certainty, only possibilities. This approach still flourishes today in many areas of academic thinking.

We will agree also that much skepticism about magnetic therapy is justified by the torrent of unfounded and exaggerated claims. Anecdotal reports without any documentation deserve to be met with a keen challenge. Consider the following:

> A forty-six-year-old man had "suffered for years from severe
> heart flutter, diarrhea, and nausea." No treatment seemed
> to help, but when a weak magnet with less than one-gauss
> strength was placed over the region of his solar plexus for
> only three minutes, his symptoms immediately ceased, and
> had never recurred on his two-year follow-up.

This came, not as you might suspect, from a magnet manufacturer on the Internet, but from a very popular, telephone directory-sized text on alternative medicine, based on the experiences of over 300 physicians and other health professionals. These alleged cases are difficult to explain or comprehend.

# Placebos

---

Another major stance for skeptics who disbelieve all the good reports about the benefits of magnetic therapy is to point at the placebo effect. If the patient believes he will get well, then he will. The word placebo comes from the Latin equivalent to "I will please." In all therapies some degree of placebo effect is present. In ancient times, healers treated the whole person who was sick or injured—both the soul and body. Sometimes a treatment would succeed when both healer and patient believed it would, even though no physical effects on the body were apparent. Today, when a new therapy or drug is tested for safety and efficacy, a major requirement is to factor out the placebo effect. Neither researcher nor subject must know which substance is the real or which the false since this knowledge would influence the results and thus destroy accuracy.

Even the most careful study always includes some allowance that the placebo effect could play a part, however small. And not every study is 100% foolproof due to yet another effect, which you might call the flip side of the placebo: what the investigators *expect* the results to be (or worse, what the investigators *want* the results to be). Physicists have long acknowledged the effect the observer has on the observed.

But, as we mentioned earlier, the placebo effect can't be trotted out to dismiss a new therapy when research involves animals or infants. These subjects could not respond solely by what is explained to them concerning what the treatment will or will not do. In the animal world, equine therapy is the prime example.

You've no doubt winced when you saw an incident in which a fine and well-loved horse was shot because its leg was broken. In recent years, veterinarians have learned that many fractures in horses can be healed with magnet therapy. Magnets are also very useful for the many hoof conditions of horses (see figure 9.1). Magnetic hoof pads treat cracking of hoof and sole, nail pricks, stone bruises, injuries to the coffin bone, thrush and seedy toe, and navicular disease. Such magnets can be worn continuously. Athletic boots protect tendons and ligaments, and hock wraps relieve pain and inflammation associated with sprains and distensions of the joint.

There are also magnetic blankets, worn over the horse's back and tied in front, to improve overall health and fitness. Used before riding, the blankets serve as warm-up preparation to enhance blood circulation, and after a competition, to prevent soreness and stiffness. As a preventive, the magnetic blanket also helps guard against ligament, tendon, muscle, or bone injury. The results have been extremely gratifying to horse owners and trainers, and no doubt to the horses themselves.

Continuing in the placebo vein: It has been proposed by a few researchers that new disorders like chronic fatigue syndrome and fibromyalgia, and symptoms of pain, weakness, and depression in other patients, may be due to depletion of magnetic energy in certain tissues, or interference with utilization. Support for this comes from anecdotal reports of marked improvement in energy levels, as well as reduction of pain and inflammation, following permanent magnet electromagnetic field therapy. Studies in animals and infants confirm that these are *not* placebo effects.

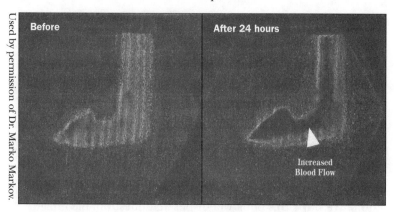

**Figure 9.1**

The images above represent the blood circulation in a horse's leg taken
before and after applying a magnet under the horse shoe.

## Further Sources of Skepticism

Money, or unfortunately the lack of it, plays a part in the slow
acceptance of magnet therapy by the scientific establishment
as a whole. Scant scientific evidence is available to support
most claims about negative-only magnetic fields healing all
across the board, and potential researchers have little financial
incentive to prove results, since they are unlikely to obtain protective patents on any discoveries.

To the best of our knowledge, only one company has
spent significant money to fund double-blind studies or establish an in-house research division headed by a qualified scientist to study how magnets work and how they can be improved.
We welcome any additional information of this nature, and
hope this book will encourage manufacturers to support scientific studies and conduct research on their products to demonstrate health benefits.

Peer pressure is another important factor to weigh in skepticism. Among all the professions, scientists, medical researchers, and physicians are particularly sensitive to peer pressure. It is not a wise career move for those on their way up the ladder to become involved in a new area that has a long battle for acceptance ahead, or for those at the top to risk their status by endorsing a fringe therapy that trails even faint clouds of quackery. This aura has plagued magnetic therapy for centuries and may now be off-putting to legitimate scientists and investigators. We hope this book will dispel that questionable image.

The skeptics' point of view may also be fueled by the uncertainty still surrounding this new therapy, as they hear magnet manufacturers argue about the virtues and safety of north versus south, unipolar versus bipolar, static versus pulsed. The more these questions remain unsettled, the more they feed the skeptical attitude.

Dr. Lawrence notes that most doctors, like most everyone, tend to put down any form of therapy with which they are unfamiliar. We fear the unknown, and unless we are enlightened on the subject, frequently allow criticism that is not justified. It's a lot like entering a dark room. We feel uneasy, but once the lights are turned on and we can see the entire room, our fear fades away and we become more comfortable in our surroundings. This is what happens when we learn about things from the bottom up, when we begin to use and observe a technique or nutrient that is new to us—we essentially learn by going where we have to go.

Perhaps a reading of the studies in this book will open the minds of a group of scientists who agree as to magnetism's effect but feel it has no therapeutic value on the body. Dr. Lawrence would like to assure them that he has learned from actual clinical experience over the last few years that magnets help in at least 80% of the conditions for which he has used them—primarily in the areas of pain relief.

A major skeptic of magnet therapy is the Federal Food and Drug Administration. So far the FDA has approved no indications for the use of permanent magnets. Sellers of magnetic devices to relieve pain are allowed to say only that they may "ease discomfort." But the consumer can figure it out.

In all fairness, some claims made by magnetic device manufacturers are far too exaggerated, especially those that claim 100% response. You won't get 100% improvement or response for *any* therapy, simply because there is too much individual biochemical difference. Every person responds differently to each treatment or medication or nutritional supplement, whether morphine or vitamin C.

How soon magnet therapy will rise to the level of acceptance that acupuncture now has gained is hard to guess. At present, anyone can make, buy, and use magnets for whatever purpose they choose. While companies are prohibited from making medical claims, including pain relief, federal regulatory agencies don't have the manpower to enforce this effectively. Consumers may be confused or misled by promotional efforts on the Internet, or by the promises of slick salespeople. And it's also difficult for consumers to distinguish between products that have good quality control and consistent gauss ratings and those that rarely deliver what they promise. Proper standards must be established and implemented to protect the public from inferior products that don't do the job. It would be a shame if the baby were thrown out with the bathwater.

However, we hope that the current research studies described at the North American Academy of Magnetic Therapy meeting and those scheduled for the future will provide enough proof to break this deadlock, and allow the freer circulation of information that confirms that magnets do relieve pain and speed healing.

A commentary by Dr. Frank Adams in the *American Journal of Pain Management,* January 1998 covered the development of an entirely magnetic approach to pain relief:

> The youthful science and practice of pain management . . . is a field still riven with internecine struggles, with specialties trumpeting ideologies over science, each claiming exclusivity to a complex clinical disorder which more often than not defeats our best efforts. We grow, and our patients ultimately benefit when we are able to transcend our petty bickering in favor of the larger issue. Another treatment option is a welcome addition to the family, and the ability to embrace, incorporate, and nurture any new idea is a sign of intellectual and clinical maturity.

Physicians and scientists would do well to remind themselves that even though human beings have learned a lot about the forces of the universe, they still have a long way to go. Albert Einstein, referring to his theory of relativity, remarked, "I can't believe that God would play dice with the universe." Danish physicist Niels Bohr is said to have replied: "It may look as if God is playing dice with the universe, but we do not have all the information God has."

So, although not all the information is in yet, scientists and researchers are seeking diligently. Until the facts have been discovered, and proved to the satisfaction of everyone (especially the skeptics), the case for magnet therapy is open to debate. That could last a long time; we hope this delay will not prevent this valuable therapy from reaching those millions who could benefit.

We remind all skeptics of the popular saying: "If it ain't broke, don't fix it." When it comes to magnetic therapy, we propose this response: "If it works, don't knock it."

# CHAPTER 10

# Serendipity and Science

*The scientist does not study nature because it is useful; he studies it because he delights in it, and he delights in it because it is beautiful. If nature were not beautiful, it would not be worth knowing, and if nature were not worth knowing, life would not be worth living.*

—Jules Henri Poincaré

The wedding between magnetism and electricity required a lengthy courtship, and the bonds of matrimony were forged by three separate events. The first was Oersted's discovery of the influence of an electric current on a magnetized needle. This demonstrated that static magnetic fields are produced by electric currents. His 1820 report of this spurred Faraday on to prove that a changing or moving magnetic field would induce an electrical current to flow in a closed circuit. The marriage contract was finally signed when Maxwell predicted that a changing electric field must have an associated magnetic field. It was sort of like a triple-play in baseball.

Let's go back and examine these episodes, because each provides an important lesson. Oersted's discovery occurred while he was demonstrating an electric current to his students and a nearby compass needle moved. Galvani was showing his electrical machine to some friends, when an assistant's scalpel touched the nerve of a skinned frog to be used for soup. As the muscles of the frog leg suddenly and unexpectedly contracted, Galvani's wife noted that a spark had been produced by the machine and "fancied that there was an agreement in point of time." A subsequent laboratory accident led Galvani to discover that two dissimilar metals completing a circuit would do the same thing. All three fortuitous accidents are sometimes referred to as examples of serendipity, or "the faculty of making lucky discoveries."

The word serendipity was coined in 1754 by Horace Walpole, who adopted it from "The Three Princes of Serendip." This was the title of a fairy tale whose leading characters "were always making discoveries by accidents and sagacity, of things that they were not in quest of." Serendipity really does not apply to Oersted or Galvani, or for that matter, Newton's observation of a falling apple. To recognize the implications of what they had observed took a lot more than just dumb luck. These were all inquisitive scientists who were well primed, so that these "accidents" merely pulled the trigger of a loaded gun. Remember Pasteur's admonition: "Chance favors the prepared mind."

The lesson to learn from Michael Faraday is much more important, since it anticipates the real message of this chapter. Faraday always firmly believed in what he referred to as "the unity of the forces of nature." What he meant by this was the conviction that all the forces of nature were really different manifestations of some single, unknown universal force. Therefore, a logical conclusion to him was that any one force ought to be convertible into any other. That's the reason he was able to quickly design an ingenious experiment to prove that if an electric current could create a magnetic field, the reverse also must be true.

In 1846, Faraday was asked to suddenly replace a speaker who failed to show up before a packed house at the Royal Institution. The lecture was to have been one of a series designed to educate the public about scientific advances. Faraday had nothing prepared, but on the spur of the moment, decided he would entitle his impromptu presentation "Thoughts on Ray Vibrations." This allowed him to review how he came to invent the term "magnetic field" by visualizing the existence of field or flux lines around a magnet. Consistent with his views of the unity of nature, he argued that there must be similar fields in the universe, as he had already shown for electricity. He then turned his attention to atoms, which were believed to be the smallest particles in nature. If there was unity in nature, then possibly the lines of electric and magnetic force associated with atoms was the medium by which light waves were propagated. This was an outlandish proposal, and there was no way Faraday, who was trained as a chemist, could even attempt to prove it. However, many years later, James Clerk Maxwell did.

# Maxwell Sees the Light
# and Hertz Helps to Shine It

Maxwell's discovery confirmed Faraday's faith in the unity of forces, and he searched for other ways to prove that all matter must exhibit some response to a magnetic field. He eventually was able to demonstrate this by following a peculiar path. He discovered that some elements (such as iron, nickel, cobalt, and oxygen) lined up in a magnetic field so that the long axis of their molecular structure was parallel to the lines of force. However, others lined up in a perpendicular arrangement. Substances in the first group were attracted to more intense magnetic fields, while those in the second moved toward regions of less magnetic force. Faraday described the first group as being paramagnetic, and named the second diamagnetic. He wondered what purpose this difference served, since Nature must have had some reason for this. He found that paramagnetics conducted magnetic lines of force better than the surrounding medium, whereas diamagnetics conducted them less well. By 1850, Faraday had developed a totally new concept of space and force.

Space was not simply a place where matter and forces were located. It was not an empty "nothing" but rather some sort of medium that physically supported fields of electric and magnetic forces. And all of the energies in the universe were similarly not localized in the particles from which these forces came but rather in the space that surrounded them. The marriage of science and electricity had given birth to what we now call field theory, and Faraday was the obstetrician.

The pediatrician who brought the baby along was James Clerk Maxwell, a Scottish physicist who was strongly influenced by Faraday's research. He thought he could prove the validity of this radical theory by translating these experimental findings into mathematical expressions, and synthesize electricity and magnetism into one coherent electromagnetic theory. He proposed that electrical energy was in the space around conductors, as well as in the conductors themselves. By 1864 he had drawn up his electromagnetic theory that incorporated light and wave phenomena into electromagnetism. He predicted that electric and magnetic fields traveled together through space as waves of electromagnetic radiation, and that light was simply one example of this. His complicated explanation for his theory has now been reduced to four elegant equations that physics students wear on T-shirts, like Einstein's $e = mc^2$. Maxwell's equations showed that light traveled at a speed of 186,000 miles per second, and according to this prediction, so would everything else in the electromagnetic spectrum. They differ from each other only in the frequency at which their electric and magnetic fields oscillate.

But the lesson we need to learn is not that Maxwell was the first person to really "see the light." What is significant is that, although nobody could disprove the logic of his mathematics, Maxwell's contemporaries refused to accept the notion that light was simply one of possibly several manifestations of electromagnetic energy. The leading authorities of the day made the following comments on Maxwell's work:

**Lord Kelvin:** "I may say one thing about it. I don't think it is admissible."

**Sir Richard Glazebrook:** "A somewhat gross conception."

**Max Planck:** "Found no foothold in Germany and was scarcely even noted."

In the beautiful quotation that began this chapter, Henri Poincaré suggests that he would particularly appreciate Maxwell's attempt to show some unity in nature. He was a brilliant French mathematician who had developed differential equations to explain the mathematics of planetary orbits, and also believed that there was a universal force and purposeful design in nature. He would surely have been sympathetic, if not supportive. However, he described his reaction as "a feeling of uneasiness, often even of mistrust, is mingled with admiration."

It was not until 1886 that Maxwell was vindicated, when the German physicist Heinrich Hertz verified the existence of electromagnetic waves traveling at the speed of light. The waves he discovered are now known as radio waves. Hertz made lots of other discoveries and contributions, one of the most important being an overhaul and simplification of Maxwell's complicated mathematical formulations into four equations. Otherwise, physics students would be walking around with mathematical expressions all over the front, back, and sides of their T-shirts.

## "Magnetism Is the King of All Secrets."

It was subsequently shown that radio, television, infrared rays, ultraviolet light, x-rays, and gamma rays all travel through space at the same speed as light, since they differ from each other only in the frequency at which their electric and magnetic fields oscillate. All waves have a wave length, which is the distance between their crests. The crests of waves in the ocean may be twenty to thirty feet apart, while sound wavelengths vary in inches. Electromagnetism also comes in waves. What distinguishes the above components of the electromagnetic spectrum is simply their wavelength. Visible light (blue, green, orange, red) is in the middle of the spectrum; radio and microwaves have longer wavelengths; and ultraviolet, x-ray, and gamma rays have shorter ones.

Remember that, although we still use Maxwell's equations to explore outer space today, his theories were not accepted in his day. People tend to reject change, especially when they can't comprehend the new concept. The first subatomic particle, the electron, was discovered only 100 years ago, because of an improved understanding of the nature of magnetic fields. In 1905, Albert Einstein's special theory of relativity established beyond a doubt that electricity and magnetism are aspects of one common phenomenon. During the late 1960s, physicists discovered that two other forces in nature have fields with a mathematical structure similar to that of the electromagnetic field and gravity. These are the strong nuclear forces responsible for the energy released in nuclear fusion, and the weak nuclear force exhibited in the radioactive decay of unstable atomic nuclei.

Just like Faraday, physicists have been trying to integrate all four forces into one grand unified theory. They have not been successful. Many believe that a fifth force will prove to be the glue that holds everything together. Some conceive of it as an energy like *Qi*, which is increasingly being acknowledged but is still poorly understood. Claims for various nutrients, electromagnetic devices, and even magnet applications that fortify "bioenergy" or trap it from the atmosphere (like Reich's orgone box) abound, are unsupported, and are sometimes pure hype.

No wonder responsible investigators like Bob Becker, Edgar Mitchell *(The Way of the Explorer)*, Bill Tiller *(Science and Human Transformation)*, Wolfgang Ludwig, and Richard Gerber *(Vibrational Medicine)* are sometimes lumped in with such dreamers and derided. Because this is an area which, like extrasensory perception and *psi* phenomena, we just don't understand, it would be wise to remember Maxwell's story. You will shortly see that good evidence exists to show that permanent magnet fields are similar to or can influence this inner energy, and provide important clues about its nature. As Paracelsus wrote, "Magnetism is the king of all secrets."

# The Flying Frog

And we seem to be uncovering more about magnetism each day. Several years ago, Japanese scientists created a magnetic compound composed only of carbon, hydrogen, nitrogen and oxygen, ingredients found in caffeine, and tons of other chemicals that have biologic effects. Unfortunately, to demonstrate significant magnetic properties, it was necessary to cool things down to almost absolute zero. That problem has now been solved. Researchers recently rearranged the constituents in caffeine and Prussian blue dye to produce two entirely new kinds of magnets. They are actually easier to make than metal ones, and are also lighter and more flexible. One contains a compound consisting of an organic molecule and vanadium, which is a nonmagnetic metal.

Although it's not likely that a magnet will cause caffeine to jump up from your coffee, it's not inconceivable that we may have blueprints that stick to a refrigerator door. The reason they work is that their atoms are arranged in rigid lattices that tighten interactions between electrons that encourage them to align their spin. Chemists believe they can manipulate this even further to produce organic magnets that will rival metal ones at even higher temperatures, and some already stick to things at

108°. It's important to emphasize that magnetism is not a property of metals per se, but of their spin, which causes them to act like tiny magnets with a north and south pole. If you can get the electrons in anything to spin so that more of these poles face in the same direction, that thing will become a magnet.

One unusual feature of some nonmetallic magnets is that their properties change when they are exposed to light. Because they weigh so little and bend so easily, nonmetallic coatings may be far superior to the flexible magnetic coatings currently used to make audio- and videotapes and optical data storage systems. This is being intensively investigated. The inventor of one nonmetallic type indicated that a manufacturer of cosmetics had contacted him, although he doesn't know why. So did a doctor hoping to improve the magnetic valves in hearts. Here's something else that would have amazed old Gilbert. You can't pick up a block of ruthenium with a magnet. But scientists recently predicted that if you put just one atomic layer of this platinum-like element on a neutral substrate, it will become as magnetic as a block of iron. Thus, it is quite possible to create magnetism where it never existed before.

We haven't talked much about gravity, but Dr. Rosch believes that studying permanent magnet fields may tell us a lot about this and other strange geomagnetic forces. We've all heard stories about Indian mystics who could levitate, or lift themselves off the ground at will, by somehow counteracting the force of gravity. Most people don't believe this any more than they believe myths about flying carpets, or Mohammed's flying coffin. It has been possible to levitate things with magnetic fields at extremely low temperatures not compatible with life. Of course, astronauts are weightless and float around once they are outside of the earth's gravitational surface, and our space program is important to study the effects of weightlessness on growth and other physiologic activities.

In late 1998, NASA is sending 77-year-old Senator John Glenn back into outer space on a 10-day shuttle flight to evaluate the problems of muscle loss and sleep disturbances, and the effects of various medications he will be given during the mission. However, it's not necessary to travel to outer space to study the physical and biologic effects of weightlessness. You can examine how crystals and plants grow in the absence of gravity by doing the experiments inside a magnet. And the ability to levitate does not depend on the size of the object. High field magnets have now been made that can levitate animals, and even people. Sounds dangerous, but it's not. As we have emphasized before, there is no evidence that such static or motionless magnetic fields have any harmful effects on living organisms. MRI studies use magnetic fields with strengths of 160,000 gauss (16 tesla) without causing any harm. This is powerful enough to levitate small animals.

A living frog was levitated in a magnetic field of 160,000 gauss by researchers from the Nijmegen High Field Magnet Laboratory in The Netherlands (see page 184). They report that the frog seemed quite comfortable inside the magnet, and, "afterwards, happily joined its fellow frogs in a biology department." This picture attracted a lot of interest and questions when it appeared on the Internet. How could a magnet make a frog seem to fly? Their explanation was complicated and included complex mathematical formulae, but a simple version went something like the following. Everything we refer to as matter in the universe is made up of atoms, which contain even smaller electrons that circle in an orbit around its nucleus. If you place something in a magnetic field, these electrons which are happily doing their usual thing don't like it very much, because there is a tug that tries to pull them in a different direction.

Nature tends to resist change, and there are numerous examples of this. Over the hundreds of thousands of years of human evolution, nature has developed exquisite responses so we can instantly and automatically maintain homeostasis when threatened by change. Whenever you try to disturb something that is well established, you will always meet resistance. That's not only a principle in physics established by Isaac Newton, but was illustrated by Maxwell, and is apparent with people in daily life all the time.

The electrons circling around atoms also resist attempts to disturb their usual orbits, so they create their own magnetic field. As a result, the atoms behave like little magnetic needles, all of which point in a direction opposite to the field which is being applied. You can feel this resistance effect if you try to push the two north or south poles of a strong magnet together. Imagine what it would feel like if you tried to do it with the magnets up to 1,000 times more powerful! What would happen to something that was in between these two opposing fields? In the case of the floating frog, its atoms act as tiny magnets, with a field of about 2 gauss. Not very strong, but it would still cause a compass needle to move.

These atomic magnets are repelled by the large magnet, and the force, which is directed upward, is strong enough to counteract the effect of gravity, which wants to pull them downward. As a result, the frog doesn't feel the tug of gravity, and can float around just like an astronaut in outer space. Is it possible that some people can generate enough internal energy to line their atoms up to do the same thing? Accomplished yogis and other mystics seem able to do some strange things, like go into a state of suspended animation where their heart rate and other vital signs are maintained at such low levels for so long that it is difficult to see how they stay alive. If they can walk on fiery coals, lie on beds of needles, or have needles thrust through parts of their body and instantly stop any bleeding that may result, who knows? And how do messages get from their brain to the particular part of the body that is being affected? Could it be through energy fields in the body that we know little about?

# What Is Energy?

Exactly what is energy? Where does it come from? Where does it go? For primitive man, energy was in the wind, the running water of rivers, fire, or bursts of lightning. These were forces in motion that could be seen or felt. There was also a curious and invisible type of energy that made it possible for living things to move, or plants and trees to grow. We tend to think of energy in terms of electricity, or the various ways it can be harnessed to provide light, heat, cold, and perform mechanical work. Indeed, the term "energy" is ultimately derived from *érgon,* a Greek word meaning "work." The addition of prefix *en-* (meaning "at") was the basis of *enérgeio,* a noun used by Aristotle to conjure up the image of something moving, or being active, which is kinetic energy.

However, energy also includes the capacity for doing work, or potential energy, which can exist in many different forms that have no visible motion, like a compressed spring or battery. *This coincides with Faraday's view that all forces, heat, light, and electricity, are unified and can be converted back and forth into each other, or into mechanical energy that is either kinetic or potential.* We also know that energy can neither be created or destroyed, only transformed into some other form, and that during this process, some of it is "lost" with respect to doing the required work. That's why you can't have perpetual motion, although Peter Peregrinus tried to do it with lodestone spheres, and a perpetual motion machine was built using magnets that would allegedly keep going by taking advantage of the force of gravity.

All the energy on earth is derived from the sun, including the invisible energy responsible for the life and health of all living things. The difference between cells and systems that are alive and healthy, and those that are dead or sick, is their ability to do work, or their level of energy. As indicated, the energy that is free for any activity the cell needs to do is stored in a remarkable compound called ATP. It is sometimes referred to as the "free energy of Gibbs," in honor of the great American physicist, Josiah W. Gibbs, who developed the concept of chemical potential energy. Gibbs was considered by our friend Maxwell to be the greatest theoretical physicist of his time, and had a great influence on Einstein as well. It's important that you understand what free energy is, because this may help explain how magnets work, and why they can provide so many different health benefits.

## Let's Take a Roller Coaster Ride

Einstein explained free energy by using the example of a roller coaster car. As the car ascends the first steep rise, it acquires potential energy as it progressively resists the force of gravity, and this becomes maximal at the top of the loop. When it accelerates back toward earth, this stored potential energy is constantly being converted into kinetic energy, the energy of movement. As the car ascends the second upward incline, its kinetic energy is again transformed back into potential energy, and this sequence of events is repeated over and over with each successive loop. If the transfer back and forth between kinetic and potential energy was always absolutely complete, then the car would always attain the same height on the ascending loop, and the same speed during its descent, and we would indeed have perpetual motion.

However, we all know that this does not happen because of friction between the wheels of the car and the rails, which creates heat. Although heat is a form of energy, it can't be used to help the car do its work, and therefore is dissipated back into the environment and the car eventually stops. The roller coaster car keeps going because of electricity, which supplies free energy to the system that it can use any way it wants. It can provide light or heat to any area, make the car go faster, slower, backwards, and so on. You could push the car to make it move, but you couldn't provide heat or light so that kind of energy is not free for any purpose.

Remember that ATP, which is formed in the mitochondrial powerhouse of every living cell, provides free energy to use just like we use electricity for so many different things. So, if you increase deficient ATP, you can restore sick nerve cells, heart cells, muscle cells, or any cell in the body. It's clear that electromagnetic energies can do this. Drs. Markov, Pilla, and others have now shown that permanent magnet fields can also influence the enzyme systems involved in making ATP. In addition, they could also show that the energy from *Qigong* healers had the same effect. What was intriguing was their observation that you could block the effect of the permanent magnet field by putting up a barrier, but the barrier did not stop *Qi* energy. Is magnetic force similar to *Qi* circulating through meridian pathways in the body? Remember that the ancient Chinese seemed to think so, and advocated lodestones as well as needles at acupuncture points. Learning how magnets relieve pain may thus also provide important information about how acupuncture works.

Various herbal preparations were also considered important for maintaining and replenishing *Qi*, and are still often used in conjunction with acupuncture. The sun increases ATP in plants through photosynthesis, during which chlorophyll converts its light photons to build up high-energy phosphate bonds. That's how we get our energy from foods. Could some foods increase the power of magnets? There is a fascinating study about to be published of fifty patients with physician-diagnosed and well-documented fibromyalgia and chronic fatigue syndrome. All had been taking various types of nutritional supplements, antidepressants, and analgesics for months, without any sustained benefits. Their symptoms and physical findings were carefully rated, and a new product containing basic saccharides that improve cell communication by binding to proteins and lipids on cell membranes was then added to these different daily regimens. When reevaluated at nine months, patients experienced a remarkable reduction in fatigue, aches and pains, anxiety and depression, sleep difficulties, memory loss, and almost all other symptoms. Could this be due to enhanced ATP effects? Dr. Colbert also reported significant improvement in fibromyalgia using magnets. Might adding appropriate nutrients enhance the benefit of magnet therapy even more?

The same may hold true for homeopathy. This is another alternative medicine approach that has experienced a marked surge in popularity over the past decade. Like acupuncture and magnet therapy, nobody knows how it works, and it also suffers from a lack of standardization, regulation, and scientific credibility. It is not generally appreciated that Samuel Hahnemann, the physician who founded homeopathy, had a strong interest in magnetism and its healing potential. Could there be some connection between the ability of minute dilutions of homeopathic preparations to cure and their magnetic properties? At one of the Montreux Congresses, Jacques Bienveniste presented his research on "memory" in water, which suggests this is plausible. Learning how magnets work may also help to explain much about homeopathy by providing us with a better understanding of the power of resonance, and how it relates to magnetism in water.

# Or a Ride on a Swing

Quantum physics teaches us that at subatomic levels, there is no difference between energy and matter, and that all things resonate, but do so at different frequencies. Resonance may also be important for us to understand how magnets can have such different effects. We know that neodymium, samarium, cobalt, and some other rare elements can markedly increase the strength of a magnet, but could they also provide different biologic effects? Experience with at least one electromagnetic device strongly supports this contention.

Professor Wolfgang Ludwig, who has been doing research in this area for the past thirty years in Germany, has invented several electromagnetic instruments. At the 1997 Montreux

Congress, he reported on his latest and most successful model, which is used to relieve pain and reduce stress. It contains an iron core that has been treated with sixty-two trace elements. By varying the electrical input, he is able to produce magnetic fields which oscillate at frequencies of 3, 7.8, or 20 cycles per second. Ludwig believes that these resonate with and can energize different structures in the body. Clinical results that Dr. Ludwig obtained in Germany, which were confirmed by others in the U.K., are impressive. He is applying for FDA approval of the model here.

The ancient Greeks believed there were only four elements; in medieval times, it was known that at least seven existed. By the beginning of this century, close to ninety had been identified, all shown to have magnetic properties. Now we recognize 112. They occur in certain groups or families in a mathematical fashion that has allowed scientists to predict that certain new elements would be found. Why is this so? What is the purpose of some of these esoteric elements, all of which resonate at different frequencies? We saw that an atomic layer of one called ruthenium could make anything else magnetic, even though a permanent magnet will not stick to a block of it. Strange stuff, probably because of something to do with resonance.

Resonance occurs in mechanical, acoustic, and electrical systems, and explains how a little energy goes a long way. You learned it very quickly as a kid on a swing, when you discovered you could go much faster and higher if you pulled on the ropes and kicked at just the right time. Or if you were pushing someone else, a little shove just when the swing reached the top got great results (but not if you did it a second before), and applying that push lower on the upswing would have the reverse effect.

Resonance explains how singers can shatter a glass several feet away, if the note they create is the same resonance frequency as the glass. The collapse of the Tacoma suspension bridge at Puget Sound in 1940 was caused by wind-excited vibrations that coincided with the bridge's resonance frequency. When the steps of marching soldiers resonate at the natural frequency of a bridge, it will collapse. Scientists say that even the little lapping of ocean waves can produce a force large enough to crack an iceberg. Charles Darwin's son calculated that a sympathetic vibration of the earth's natural frequency and the solar tides around four billion years ago could have ejected the moon from our ocean basin. Nikola Tesla, the electrical wizard we didn't get a chance to meet, said he could use resonance to split the world. Resonance is powerful stuff.

As Dr. Rosch has written elsewhere, in addition to being a protective shield, the cell wall must now be viewed as a powerful signal amplifier that resonates, and governs the flow of ions into and out of the cell by minute changes in electrical tension. We now know that feeble electromagnetic forces can have profound influences on cellular growth and function that do not appear to involve any heat exchange (thus violate the laws of thermodynamics). It therefore seems plausible that similar subtle energies generated internally might exert analogous effects. Thus, EEG, ECG, and EMG waves may not merely reflect the noise of the machinery of the brain, heart, and muscle; but rather reflect signals being sent to other parts of the body, or even externally. Some of these pathways and mechanisms are just beginning to be delineated.

This emerging model of communication at a physical/atomic, rather than the current chemical/molecular paradigm, helps to explain a variety of widely acknowledged but poorly understood phenomena, such as the placebo effect, the power of a strong faith in spontaneous remission of cancer, the salubrious effects of strong social support, and numerous psychokinetic observations ranging from the power of nonphysical "therapeutic touch" to the ability of *Qigong* energies to affect enzyme reactions in a test tube that are involved in energy formation in the body. Electromagnetic radiations at certain frequencies can excite atoms to higher energy levels while they remain unaffected by greater frequencies that are nonresonant.

Resonance can be a crucial factor in all of the above, and may be equally important for understanding how magnets work. It can also be used to measure minute amounts of elements in material. MRI depends on principles of nuclear magnetic resonance imaging. A patient is placed inside a cylinder that contains a strong magnet, and radio waves are then introduced, which cause the atoms of the body to resonate. Each type of body tissue resonates differently, and emits characteristic signals from the nuclei of its atoms. A computer translates these signals into a two-dimensional picture. MRI does not use ionizing radiation, does not require radioactivity labeled dyes, can see through bone, and produce images of blood vessels, cartilage, muscles, ligaments, and even bone marrow and cerebrospinal fluid. All because of resonance.

# Music, Medicine, and Mathematics

Resonance was discovered by Pythagorus over 2,500 years ago, when he found that vibrating strings only produced harmonious tones when the ratios of the length of the strings were whole numbers from one to four. If one string was exactly twice the length of another, the resultant tone would be one octave higher, 3:2 would sound together in a perfect fifth,

4:3 would create a fourth, and so on. He found the same thing in wind instruments, and centuries later, the construction of an organ pipe followed this principle. Pythagorus was an accomplished mathematician whose theorem about right-angle triangles still bears his name. Based on his knowledge of music, mathematics, and astronomy, Pythagorus was convinced that all of nature was governed by mathematical laws of harmonious proportions. He proposed that ratios of the distances between the sun, moon, and planets that he knew about would follow mathematical rules similar to those he discovered for the harmonies in music. He also believed that these huge celestial bodies created harmonious sounds as they moved through the heavens; this he called "the music of the spheres."

It was not until the seventeenth century that this concept of celestial order and harmony was confirmed by Newton and Kepler, as Robert Fludd tried to portray in his "cosmic monochord"(see page 183). Pythagorus was the first to propose that the earth was a sphere and in motion in accordance with cosmic unity.

Pythagorus was a physician; he believed that if you could understand the microcosm of music, you could heal people who were sick. He established facilities for this. The Musical Resonance Therapy of Peter Hubner is based on the same concept, and has been shown in scientific studies to increase immune system resistance to cancer and infections, and to significantly decrease pain, stress, and length of stay in hospitalized patients. At the Montreux Congress, a presentation by Fabien Maman showed how exposure to a tone of a certain frequency for 15–20 minutes would invigorate healthy cells, but cause cancerous ones to expand and explode. We all know how martial music with certain beats can be stimulating, while other music can "soothe a savage breast." At the 1998 Winter Olympics, one could see how people of all nationalities were moved by a Japanese rendition of Schiller's *Ode to Joy* from Beethoven's Ninth Symphony, even if they didn't understand the words.

Resonance is responsible not only for the sound of music, but possibly the biologic effects of other subtle energies. Electromagnetic fields promote fracture healing, but so do ultrasound waves. And it has been recently shown that shining a light on the back of the knee can influence circadian rhythms, just like melatonin. Resonance is also behind everything from the color of autumn leaves to the rings of Saturn.

# We Are Not Alone in the Universe!

*A human being is part of the whole, called by us "universe," limited in time and space. He experiences himself, his thoughts and feelings as something separated from the rest—a kind of optical delusion of his consciousness. This delusion is a prison, restricting us to our personal desires and to affection for a few persons close to us.*

*Our task must be to free ourselves from our prison by widening our circle of compassion to embrace all humanity and the whole of nature in its beauty.*

—Albert Einstein

Life on earth evolved under geomagnetic fields and electromagnetic forces that have been fairly constant for hundreds of millions of years. All that changed a little over 100 years ago, when Thomas Edison built the first power station in New York City. You can sit now in a room or some place where there is complete silence, and, with the right detectors, you can pick up AM and FM radio, television waves, electrical and magnetic fields, and other ambient pollution that results in cacophony. There is good reason to believe that many of these can affect mood and behavior, as well as biological processes. This is something new for mankind, and we do not know what the long-term effects will be. In addition to adding new forces, we are also paying less and less attention to the old ones.

We know little about the subtle subterranean energy currents that the ancient Chinese called the lines of the dragon force. These wind along the earth's surface in no particular way and vary with geographical locations. Lost civilizations were able to detect and trace these, so that they could mold the landscape to their patterns, and mark their course by temples, and mounds of stone, or other objects that would identify this natural source of power. There is evidence of this in Europe, the Middle East, Central and South America, and the Orient. In ancient Britain, the landscape was modified by erecting mounds and massive stones, and cutting notches in the skyline. The eroded traces of this can still be seen in nearly every part of the country. Dragon lines, referred to in England as ley lines, were traced by the dowser with a divining rod made of hazel. Wellsprings of water hundreds of feet beneath the surface of the earth can be detected, and dowsing is still often used today for this and other purposes. Satellite detectors confirm that there can be significant gravitational fluctuation in certain geographic areas; and in addition to water, large accumulations of quartz and other minerals can influence electromagnetic fields in overlying areas.

Chinese dragon lines were never straight, and they undulate to provide a balance of earth energy. When straight modern roads and railway lines were built, there was much opposition—because these destroy nature, and introduce unbalanced forces into the environment that make it less healthy. What is this dragon force energy? It's not electricity, and the best anyone can say is that it seems to correspond to *Qi* or *chi*. Just like meridians can trace energy paths in the body, the dragon lines seem to do this for the earth, although in neither case does it mean that these lines conduct electricity like wires. *Qi* simply seems to manifest itself in electrical terms as one aspect of its complex nature.

The ancient Chinese were aware of these patterns of environmental energy flow through a form of geomancy, called *feng* ("wind water"). They used this to determine the best site for a home or work area, what direction to sleep in, and where to place various objects to achieve the most harmonious relationships. It may sound like nonsense to some, but it is still taken very seriously by many. An article in the January 28, 1988, issue of *The Wall Street Journal* describes how bad the *feng shui* was in the "glass-walled towers of Hong Kong's Lippo Center, a giant office complex." A tycoon who bought it in 1988 went bankrupt in four years. The building was purchased by a Japanese realty company that was forced to sell it after a brief period because of financial problems. Then in 1991, a bank that had its local headquarters there collapsed in a financial scandal, and a financial firm that rented two floors the following year has recently gone under because of heavy debt.

This occurred despite the fact that the owners had their own *feng-shui* consultant check it out, and never actually moved in since they rented it to others. However, they did inscribe their name in gold letters in the lobby. A professional *feng-shui* consultant said that the building had "the worst *feng shui*" because of the large, C-shaped bulges on the sides of each office tower. Although some think these are attractive and look like giant Koala bears, he said they resembled ancient Chinese handcuffs that radiated bad luck, and "You just have to put

your name on the building, and it affects you." A skeptical ten-
ant on another floor said that although he doesn't believe in
any of this, he's hiring his own expert and says, "If he suggests
that I put in a fish tank or a small tree, I'll do that."

# There's Something in the Air
# and "The Spark of Life"

Maxwell showed that space was not empty, even before we had
electromagnetic pollution. But that notion did not originate
with him. Ancient Greeks and others believed that a fifth element permeated all of space and was a purer form of fire and
air than that of which the stars and comets were made. The
Ancient Greeks and Maxwell both referred to it as "the ether."
The ether contained the stuff of which life was made, and later
on, was believed to contain God's spirit. Coptic priests still
breathe air into all babies when they are born to transmit this
"ether" to them. We get it when we breathe in or inspire.

Children are enthusiastic when they learn they have a little of God in them *(en theos)*. In his *Principia* (1687) Isaac Newton wrote of "a certain most subtle spirit which pervades and
lies hid in all gross bodies," and that "all sensation is excited,
and the members of animal bodies move at the command of
the will, namely, by the vibrations of this spirit, mutually propagated along the solid filaments of the nerves, from the outward
organs of sense to the brain, and from the brain into the muscles." Michelangelo's depiction of this ether on the ceiling of
the Sistine Chapel shows Adam being animated by what
appears to be a spark of lightning from God's finger. Medieval
portrayals of creation, or divine healing, often showed similar

rays also emanating from the heavens, but from some un-known source. It was something in the air like electricity that gave life, and Frankenstein needed lightning.

William Gilbert thought that whatever strange force existed in magnets was the key to life. He stated: "The magnetic force is animate, or imitates a soul; in many respects it surpasses the human soul while it is united to an organic body." And it looks like electricity is involved if you want to create life by cloning something. What the Scottish investigators did was to cause cells to go into a state of rest or hibernation, during which the active genes are switched off to keep the cells from dividing. The nucleus of an unfertilized ovum is removed and attempts are made to join the cell with another containing a different nucleus. However, nothing happens unless a very gentle electrical impulse is applied, which causes them to fuse together like soap bubbles.

Successive electrical pulses then prompt the egg to accept the new nucleus as if it were its own, and also trigger a burst of biochemical activity, which then jump-starts the process of cell division. This is accomplished by putting two electrodes on the glass slide and running a very tiny current through them for a few thousandths of a second. This starts the cell on the path of dividing, very similar to that which occurs after a sperm penetrates an egg, which includes a surge of calcium and a burst of enzyme activity—literally, a "spark of life."

## Nothing New Under the Sun

*What is history after all? History is facts which become lies in the end; legends are lies which become history in the end.*

–Jean Cocteau

## Serendipity and Science

*That men do not learn very much from the lessons of history, is the most important of all the lessons that history has to teach.*

–Aldous Huxley

*The development of human thought and achievement, as a whole, has not been, as is commonly supposed, a continual upward progression, nor even the equivalent of a continuous series of ascertained results. . . . The intuition of the true investigator and pathfinder of today and tomorrow must find its own way to new guiding principles from the work of yesterday, before yesterday, and the distant path.*

–Karl Sudhoff

*And there is no new thing under the sun.*

–Ecclesiastes 1:9

Today, appeals to return to "natural" therapies appear in various Internet promotions for alternative medicine. We have added various quotations to support the view that we often "discover" things that were well appreciated long ago. Scientific progress does not necessarily occur in linear fashion with orderly progressive steps, but advances in spurts. Sometimes we take a step in the wrong direction or backward, and things that are new are not necessarily better. And sometimes things turn out not to be as crazy as they seem.

Galen wrote that women who had too much black bile (Gr. *mélas, chole*) and were melancholy were much more likely to develop cancer of the breast and uterus. Dr. Rosch, who has written extensively about relationships between stress and cancer, says Galen was absolutely right, since numerous studies confirm that women who are depressed have much higher rates of these malignancies. It has been shown that depression can lower immune system resistance to cancer, which may help to explain this. In chapter 2 we referred to promotional claims that magnets attached to your garden hose could neutralize the harmful chemicals found in water, making your plants and crops grow faster and bigger, and that other magnetic devices would prevent corrosive damage to metallic pipes or improve the taste of wine. Magnets in wells *are* used to soften water and prevent corrosion. When water moves through a magnetic field, the hydrogen ions and dissolved minerals become charged, causing molecular clusters that improve taste and make it "soft." Well water and running streams are naturally charged by the earth's 0.5-gauss magnetic field. But during water treatment and transport through city water pipes, the charge dissipates. Look at the tremendous recent increase in sales of bottled water from natural sources all over the world. Electromagnetic fields are now also being utilized to make orchids grow faster and better, and some *Qigong* masters can change the taste of scotch and wine.

Research over the past few years has shown that electromagnetic fields do produce spectacular results in patients with far-advanced cancer that has failed to respond to conventional treatment. At the same time, there are also concerns that electromagnetic fields can cause cancer. Is it a question of dosage, length of exposure, or the type of magnetic energy? Who knows? And why should it be surprising that electromagnetic energy can be a two-edged sword? X-rays, hormones, and everything else we use to treat cancer can also cause it. Chemotherapy is a mainstay of treatment, but when these drugs are given to patients to prevent rejection of heart or kidney transplants, up to 20% of recipients can develop cancer within five years. Gilbert was confused when some respected authorities said that magnets were good for hot conditions, while others insisted just the opposite. Maybe they were both right.

Much is not known. We still don't know how an electrical force gets from here to there. Perhaps, as is proposed by Richard Feynman, it is by the exchange between charged particles of quanta of electromagnetic radiation. Another unsolved problem is: What holds an electron together? Quantum physicists say that a negative charge on one side repelling the negative charge on the other side would tear the particle apart. Some strange attractive force must be involved; and although a fifth force has been postulated many times, it has not been found. Could *Qi* be the glue? Could magnets hold the key to this? Remember what Paracelsus said: "Magnetism is the king of all secrets."

It's clear that we have yet to discover most of the magnet's secrets. There are surely many more questions than answers. Nobody has proven that one kind of magnet is better than another for pain relief or other problems. Some may be stronger, but this may not always mean better. We don't know how strong a magnet needs to be for any application, but we know you don't need a howitzer to shoot down a robin. The magnetic insoles Dr. Michael Weintraub used for diabetic neuropathy were bipolar products. Would single-pole application be as good, or provide increased relief more quickly? That can only be determined by carefully designed double-blind studies, which nobody wants to fund.

In *The Structure of Scientific Revolution,* Thomas Kuhn asks "Does a field make progress because it is a science, or is it a science because it makes progress?" Up to the present, the study of magnets has been a field. It is just starting to become a science. We don't know how magnets, acupuncture, homeopathy, or for that matter, how aspirin works; but that's not particularly important. Theories don't have to be correct; only facts do. It's all very well to theorize, but it's what we *learn* from carefully conducted experiments that really counts. Some theories are valuable because of their heuristic merit, in that they encourage others to discover new facts that prove they are wrong, and ultimately lead to better theories. Orthopedist Andrew Bassett stated it well:

> In the decade to come, it is safe to predict, bioelectromag-
> netics will assume a therapeutic importance equal to, or
> greater than, that of pharmacology and surgery today.
> With proper interdisciplinary effort, significant inroads
> can be made in controlling the ravages of cancer, some
> forms of heart disease, arthritis, hormonal disorders, and
> neurological scourges such as Alzheimer's disease, spinal
> cord injury, and multiple sclerosis. This prediction is not
> pie in-the-sky. Pilot studies, and biological mechanisms
> already defined in primordial terms, form a rational basis
> for such a statement.

Andy Basset passed away a few years after he made this prophetic statement in a 1992 article. He and Bob Becker were the orthopedists who developed the only currently approved electromagnetic device, which is for healing un-united fractures. There is little doubt that he was right on target, and while he didn't live to see his prediction come true, most of you will be able to appreciate the important role of bioelectromagnetic medicine in twenty-first century medicine. It is very likely that we will soon see other approved indications for electromagnetic field therapies, and probably for permanent magnets as well.

When Paracelsus said, "Magnetism is the king of all secrets," he may have been more on target than he suspected. Faraday and Maxwell were able to construct a theory that unified electricity and magnetism, and predicted that there would be other energies in the electromagnetic spectrum such as light and radio waves. Magnetism may hold the key to understanding how other subtle energies like light, sound, aromas, therapeutic touch, massage, or *Qigong* exert their biologic and healing effects. What is the mechanism whereby music improves immune function, or shining a light on the back of the knee influences circadian rhythms? What about the weak energies that can be generated internally that may also have biologic effects? What about the role of faith, or intentionality in producing spontaneous remission in cancer and other deadly disorders? How is this accomplished? Dr. Rosch, who is on the Advisory Board of the Institute of Heart Math, points to their extensive research showing how the mind can affect heart rate variability, and how this can be used as a powerful stress reduction tool with their "Freeze-Frame" technique. How does this communication take place?

Our hope is that this book will stimulate such efforts to explain the unity of forces and the mystery and magic of magnets.

You will recall that Dr. Nordenstrom suspects that the energy flowing in his "electrical" circulatory system is probably the same as *Qi*, but that "nobody knows what *Qi* is." The ancient Chinese sage Lao Tsu described it as follows:

Look, it cannot be seen–it is beyond form
Listen, it cannot be heard–it is beyond sound
Grasp, it cannot be held–it is intangible.

He might as well have been talking about magnetism.

# CHAPTER 11

# Conclusion

## *Your Proactive Health Future*

A mid the confusion of a shifting medical paradigm, as alternative and holistic therapies begin to join mainstream medicine, you the patient (or "health consumer" as the economists would have it) need to find a solid path by seeking information and learning what all the options are. Naturally, you want the most effective, the safest, the most economical route. But you may need to become more aggressive in order to fight an often unsatisfactory health-care system for necessary treatments, and to find a qualified yet enlightened physician. This can be an uphill battle, but one well worth winning. In essence, good health is not found in the doctor's office; it starts with you.

Public opinion plays a crucial role in today's changing medical paradigm, as was evidenced in 1994 by the overwhelming public support for S.784, the Dietary Supplement Health and Education Act. Threatened with the loss of easy access to vitamins and other nutritional supplements, the public bombarded Capitol Hill with phone calls, letters, and faxes. It was the largest grass roots response in decades.

Therefore, it is quite possible that the public will lead the medical profession into recognizing the benefits of magnetic therapy by trying it themselves—before the official establishment even acknowledges its existence. The public has been increasingly distressed when therapies that appear to be safe, are effective, and have been approved in other countries that also have stringent regulations are not available in the United States.

This awareness accelerated several years ago, when *Discover* magazine published a cover story on Dr. Bjorn Nordenstrom, describing his theory of the body's electrical circulatory system as the most important advance in medicine since 1628, when William Harvey discovered how blood circulated in the body. A *20/20* television program devoted to Dr. Nordenstrom showed how he cured a patient with cancer of the lung in a 30-minute procedure that was painless, inexpensive, and did not require an overnight hospital stay. Americans are unaware, unwilling, or unable to travel to Sweden or even to China, where these results have been confirmed in thousands of patients. Nor do they go to Mexico City, where Dr. Demetrio Sodi-Pallares has had incredible results with electromagnetic therapy in treating patients with far-advanced metastatic malignancies, and those with end-stage cardiomyopathy who can't get heart transplants. Some of these patients, who would have been dead in weeks, are leading active, healthy lives two or more years later, and are on no medications.

Both these physicians, who are friends of Dr. Rosch, have impeccable credentials and have presented their research at the yearly Montreux conference. Dr. Nordenstrom headed the Department of Radiology at the Karolinska Institute in Stockholm for years, during which he originated the stereotactic technique that allows surgeons to pinpoint lesions and treat them without opening the chest or brain. He was Chairman of the Nobel Assembly and the Committee that selects the Nobel Laureate for Physiology and Medicine, and has been himself nominated for the Nobel Prize.

Dr. Demetrio Sodi-Pallares is a distinguished Mexican cardiologist who has been designated Master Teacher of the American College of Cardiology. He has written twenty books on this subject, including over a dozen on the electrocardiogram alone. He formulated the concept of the cellular sodium pump, which keeps tissue alive and healthy by maintaining the right balance between the sodium and potassium ions inside and outside of cell membranes. This led to the development, over forty years ago, of his polarizing solution for the treatment of acute heart attacks. It reduced complications and hospital stays dramatically, and is still being used to protect patients whose hearts must be stopped for extended periods during cardiac surgery. At the 1997 conference in Montreux, he presented the remarkable results he has achieved by combining electromagnetic therapy, polarizing solution, and diet for patients dying from terminal heart disease (cardiomyopathy) and cancer. He presented his early research at the annual meeting of the North American Academy of Magnetic Therapy two years ago. Both Drs. Lawrence and Rosch have sent patients with advanced cancers that have failed to respond to conventional therapy to Dr. Sodi-Pallares.

American patients who don't understand why they can't get such therapies here are not aware that it could take up to ten years and millions of dollars to go through the FDA approval process. Some critics even feel that powerful vested financial interests are keeping these new therapies out. Cancer therapy is big business. As a result of all the uproar, Congress has come down on the FDA, and passed (with little discussion) the Food and Drug Administration Act of 1997. Designed to speed things up, the Act promised to provide information on its own implementation. The first document under this Act became available (on February 6, 1998) and was issued without the customary appeal for public comment because of the desire to implement it immediately. However, comments and suggestions about these new revisions "can be submitted within 90 days to Docket No. 98D-0003."

Here is a note of hope: This new act contains language that will increase the likelihood that some permanent magnet products will now be approved by the FDA for pain relief, since they should be able to meet the revised standards. We urge those of you who have already benefited from magnetic therapy to contact your elected representatives on this matter. We will try to keep you updated if you request information via e-mail addresses for Dr. Rosch (stress124@pol.net) or Dr. Lawrence (neurodoc@pol.net). The North American Academy of Magnetic Therapy is planning to establish a Web site, but you can contact them at 800-457-1853. Information on the next Montreux Congress on Stress, which will again feature sessions devoted to the latest advances in magnetotherapy from around the world, can be obtained at http://www.stress.org.

The authors of this book hope you will become proactive in your own healing. If you have a persistent health problem that is not responding to a prescribed treatment, learn to play detective and gather clues from all possible, but credible, sources; then share this information with your doctor. If you meet a closed mind, keep searching until you find a healthcare professional who will take time to listen carefully and act as your partner.

We urged you in the Introduction to share this book with your doctor. By now you know that parts of the magnet therapy picture are quite technical. Your physician will not only understand these parts, but is likely to be motivated to learn more.

The authors do not recommend any specific product or manufacturer. Claims for superiority are based on anecdotal reports and promotional speculations. Proof must await careful correlation to determine proper dosage and duration of treatment for specific disorders. We had intended to provide a list of magnet manufacturers with toll-free numbers, but this is not feasible. Companies are springing up and going out of business all the time—many of the listings we thought were current are already defunct. Others are unable to provide anything except a price list. Let the buyer beware. Any reputable manufacturer should be willing to provide supportive references, gauss ratings for their products, and a 30-day money back guarantee. And don't expect instant results. Prompt benefits are sometimes dramatic, but it often takes days before there is significant improvement.

The full potential of magnet therapy can only be realized by proper scientific studies. It is our hope that this book will encourage such efforts by the public and private sectors, and particularly FDA-approved and sponsored protocols. Some of these may already be under way, so stay tuned.

Although one would have to say magnet therapy is still in the formative stage, its future is bright with promise—very bright indeed. One might even add that, as we are naturally attracted to healing and relief from pain, magnet therapy is pulling us irresistibly forward.

# INDEX

# Index

# Index

# *Index*

3–D distribution of magnetic fields, 175

Tibet, 7, 140

Tic douleureux, 78–79

Tiller, Bill, 199

TMJ (temporomandibular joint disorder), 96

Transcranial Magnetic Stimulation (TMS), 139–141

*Treatise on Diseases of Workers* (Ramazzini), 132

Trigeminal neuralgia, 78

Truck driver's fatigue, 146

T-shirt for shoulder pain, 103–104, 112–113

Tuberculosis, 95

Tufts Medical School, 175, 176

Tungsten, 38

Tylenol and alcohol, 63

## U

Ultraviolet, 57

Unipolar magnets, 121, 181

University of Pavia, 48

University Sleep Laboratories, 145

Urate crystals, 95

## V

Valium

for fibromyalgia, 176

Symtonic LEET and, 75

Vallbona, Carlos, 142, 153, 181

Van Kerrebroeck, 79

Van Musschenbrock, Peter, 42–43

Vardanian, 130

The Vedas, 2

Vermillion, Ryan, 102

Verschuur, 53

Vibrating, moving magnet, 123–124

Volta, Alessandro, 19, 46, 48–50, 122

Voltaic cell experiment, 53–55

## W

Walpole, Horace, 194

Washington, George, 16

Water, 124, 219

in India, 149

Weight gain, 97–98

Weightlessness, 202

Weintraub, Michael, 147, 163, 220

Whittingham, Charles, 100

Window phenomenon, 119–120

Wordsworth, William, 151

Wound healing, 129–131

case histories of, 130–131

Wraps, 112

Wrist, placement of magnets on, 111

## X

X-rays, 56, 155–156

ionizing radiation from, 156

## Y

Yellow bile, 32

*The Yellow Emperor's Book of Internal Medicine,* 2

Yin and yang, 2, 4, 5

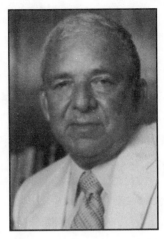

**Paul J. Rosch, M.D.,** is a fellow and life member of the American College of Physicians. An international authority on the relationship between stress and illness, he has served as president of the American Institute of Stress for 20 years. Editor of *Stress Medicine,* Dr. Rosch has written extensively on all aspects of stress over the past 45 years. He is a clinical professor of medicine and psychiatry at New York Medical College and past president of the New York State Society of Internal Medicine. He has been interviewed on *60 Minutes* and widely quoted in the media, including *Time, The Wall Street Journal, New York Times,* and *London Times.*

**Ron Lawrence, M.D., Ph.D.,** is president of the North American Academy of Magnetic Therapy. Considered a leading authority on the medical use of magnets and a respected neurologist with over 45 years experience, Dr. Lawrence established the first in-patient pain center in the United States. He has studied and practiced acupuncture, served on the National Advisory Council on Aging at the National Institute of Health, and is an assistant clinical professor at the UCLA School of Medicine. Author of several books, Dr. Lawrence has appeared on many national television programs and radio shows.

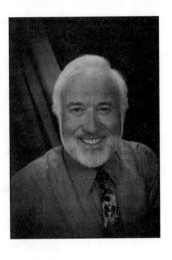

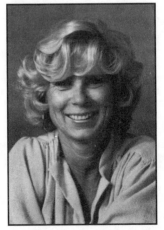

**Judith Plowden** is a professional writer based in Los Angeles. As well as being the former managing editor of the *Journal of Longevity Research,* she has sold many television and feature scripts, and is also a published novelist, poet, and the writer of *Inner Silence* (Harper & Row, 1987).

# Restore Your Body's Vital Energy

Work, stress, junk food, caffeine, colds, late nights, and all the other challenges our bodies face every day can take their toll, depleting the basic vital energy the Chinese call *chi*. Ginseng and the tonic herbs–especially when combined with changes in diet and lifestyle–can replenish depleted *chi*, restoring balance in the body, invigorating the immune system, and enhancing strength and stamina. Author Paul Bergner explains the Chinese holistic approach to health in simple terms, describing how to use ginseng and the tonic herbs for the best possible results.

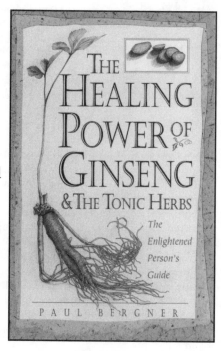

U.S. $14.95 / Can. $19.95
ISBN 0-7615-0472-9
paperback / 288 pages

# To Order Books

Please send me the following items:

| Quantity | Title | Unit Price | Total |
|----------|-------|------------|-------|
| _____ | **The Healing Power of Ginseng** | $ **14.95** | $ _____ |
| _____ | **The Natural Pharmacy** | $ **19.99** | $ _____ |
| _____ | _____ | $ _____ | $ _____ |
| _____ | _____ | $ _____ | $ _____ |
| _____ | _____ | $ _____ | $ _____ |

| *Shipping and Handling depend on Subtotal. | | |
|---|---|---|
| **Subtotal** | **Shipping/Handling** | |
| $0.00–$14.99 | $3.00 | |
| $15.00–$29.99 | $4.00 | |
| $30.00–$49.99 | $6.00 | |
| $50.00–$99.99 | $10.00 | |
| $100.00–$199.99 | $13.50 | |
| $200.00+ | Call for Quote | |

Foreign and all Priority Request orders:
Call Order Entry department
for price quote at 916-632-4400

This chart represents the total retail price of books only (before applicable discounts are taken).

|  |  |
|---|---|
| Subtotal | $ _____ |
| Deduct 10% when ordering 3—5 books | $ _____ |
| 7.25% Sales Tax (CA only) | $ _____ |
| 8.25% Sales Tax (TN only) | $ _____ |
| 5% Sales Tax (MD and IN only) | $ _____ |
| 7% G.S.T. Tax (Canada only) | $ _____ |
| Shipping and Handling* | $ _____ |
| Total Order | $ _____ |

**By Telephone:** With American Express, MC or Visa, call 800-632-8676 or 916-632-4400.   Mon–Fri, 8:30-4:30.

**WWW:** http://www.primapublishing.com

**By Internet E-mail:** sales@primapub.com

**By Mail:** Just fill out the information below and send with your remittance to:

**Prima Publishing**
**P.O. Box 1260BK**
**Rocklin, CA 95677**

Name _____

Address_____

City _____ State _____ ZIP_____

MC/Visa#_____ Exp. _____

Check/money order enclosed for $ _____ Payable to Prima Publishing

Daytime telephone _____

Signature _____